D1796667

Male Infertility
from A to Z

A concise encyclopedia

STUDIES IN PROFERTILITY SERIES

VOLUME 4

Male Infertility from A to Z

A concise encyclopedia

J.M.G.HOLLANDERS, J.A. CARVER-WARD

AND K. A. JAROUDI, E. MEULEMAN, U. V. SIECK, S. A. TOOK

*The publication of this book has been made possible
by an educational grant from NV Organon*

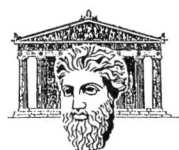

The Parthenon Publishing Group
International Publishers in Medicine, Science & Technology

NEW YORK   LONDON

Published in the USA by
The Parthenon Publishing Group Inc.
One Blue Hill Plaza
PO Box 1564, Pearl River,
New York 10965, USA

Published in the UK by
The Parthenon Publishing Group
Casterton Hall, Carnforth,
Lancs, LA6 2LA, UK

Library of Congress Cataloging-in-Publication Data

Male infertility from A to Z : a concise encyclopedia / J. M. G.
   Hollanders, J. Carver-Ward . . . [et al.]
      p.   cm. – (Studies in profertility series : v. 4)
   Includes bibliographical references.
   ISBN 1-85070-758-8
   1. Infertility, Male–Encyclopedias.   I. Hollanders, J. M. G.
   II. Series.
   RC889.M344   1996
   616.6'92'003–dc20

96-23150
CIP

British Library Cataloguing in Publication Data

Male infertility from A to Z : a concise encyclopedia. –
   (Studies in profertility series ; v. 4)
   1. Infertility, Male – Encyclopedias
   I. Hollanders, J. M. G.
   616.6'92'003

ISBN 1-85070-758-8

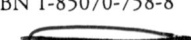

First published 1996

Composition by H&H Graphics, Blackburn, UK
Printed and bound by Butler & Tanner Ltd, Frome and London, UK

List of Authors

J.M.G. Hollanders, MD, PhD

Chairman, Department of
  Obstetrics and Gynecology
Consultant, Section of
  Reproductive Endocrinology,
  Infertility and IVF
King Faisal Specialist Hospital and
  Research Centre
PO Box 3354
11211 Riyadh
Saudi Arabia

K.A. Jaroudi, MD

Head, Section of Reproductive
  Endocrinology, Infertility and
  IVF
King Faisal Specialist Hospital and
  Research Centre
PO Box 3354
11211 Riyadh
Saudi Arabia

U.V. Sieck, MD

Consultant, Section of
  Reproductive Endocrinology,
  Infertility and IVF
King Faisal Specialist Hospital and
  Research Centre
PO Box 3354
11211 Riyadh
Saudi Arabia

J.A. Carver-Ward, MSc

Head of IVF and Andrology
Tawam Hospital
PO Box 15258
Al Ain
Abu Dhabi
United Arab Emirates

E. Meuleman, MD, PhD

Assistant Professor
Department of Urology
University Hospital Nijmegen
St Radboud
PO Box 9101
6500 HB Nijmegen
The Netherlands

S.A. Took, MD

Fellow, Section of Reproductive
  Endocrinology, Infertility and
  IVF
King Faisal Specialist Hospital and
  Research Centre
PO Box 3354
11211 Riyadh
Saudi Arabia

Electron micrograph photographs — J. McClintock

Illustrations — S.A. Ward

A*a*

ABSTINENCE PERIOD

Traditionally, the suggested optimal period for abstinence prior to giving a semen specimen for analysis has been 2–5 days. Recent literature suggests that this period is possibly 5–10 days. Volume and count increase steadily with duration of abstinence, while other parameters, including motility, morphology (Kruger's strict criteria) and hypo-osmotic swelling test, do not alter significantly. Only sperm acrosin content decrease almost twofold after 5 days of abstinence. Even for asthenozoospermic men, an increase in progressive motility after 5 days has been reported.

1. Blackwell, J.M. and Zaneveld, L.J.D. (1992). Effect of abstinence on sperm acrosin, hypoosmotic swelling, and other semen variables. *Fertil. Steril.*, **58**, 798

2. Check, J.H., Epstein, R. and Long, R. (1991). Effect of time interval between ejaculations on semen parameters. *Arch. Androl.*, **27**(2), 93–5

3. Tollefsrud, M.O., Abyholm, T. and Purvis, K. (1991). Effects of varying the abstinence period in the same individuals on sperm quality. *Arch. Androl.*, **26**(3), 199–203

Related subjects: semen analysis — normal values, collection of sample

ACQUIRED IMMUNODEFICIENCY SYNDROME (AIDS)

There is an associated impairment of male reproductive functions in patients with human immune deficiency virus infection, particularly in those with more advanced stages of the disease. This might be due to a direct effect of the virus, an HIV-related malignancy, opportunistic infections or toxic side effects of therapeutic agents for such infections. Advanced stages of the disease (AIDS related complex characterized by persistent lymphadenopathy and fever plus weight loss) are associated with a low level of testosterone and lower testosterone/ estrogen ratio. The mechanism which causes these low androgen levels is controversial, since some patients show low gonadotropins while others are hypergonadotropic. Semen analysis shows only slight variation of sperm quality, mainly reduced sperm motility, which could be related to impairment of epididymal sperm maturation following testosterone reduction. Late stages of the disease are associated with testicular atrophy. HIV positive asymptomatic patients have no significant hormonal or semen abnormalities.

1. Croxson, T.S., Chapman, W.E., Miller, L.K., Levit, C.D., Senie, R. and Zumoff, B. (1989). Changes in the hyothalamic–pituitary–gonadal axis in human immunodeficiency virus-infected homosexual men. *J. Clin. Endocrinol. Metab.*, **68**, 317

2.   Maggi, M. and Forti, G. (1994). Gonadal function in AIDS. *Bailliere's Clin. Endocrinol. Metab.*, 8(4), 849

Related subjects: human immunodeficiency virus, hypogonadotropic hypogonadism

ACROSIN

Acrosin is a serine proteinase enzyme associated with the acrosome of the spermatozoon. It is present on the inner acrosomal membrane of spermatozoa in the form of the inactive pro-acrosin. Activation of pro-acrosin during the acrosome reaction is thought to ease the binding to and the penetration of the sperm through the zona pellucida. Suspicion about deficiency of acrosin should be raised if there is no sperm binding to the zona pellucida or if no fertilization is achieved with *in vitro* fertilization (IVF).

1.   Rogers, B.J. and Bentwood, B. (1982). Capacitation, acrosome reaction and fertilization. In Zaneveld, L.J.D. and Chatterton, T.R. (eds.) *Biochemistry of Mammalian Reproduction.* (New York: John Wiley & Sons)

2.   van der Ven, H.H., Kennedy, W.P., Kaminski, J.M., Jeyendran, R.S. and Zaneveld, L.J.D. (1987). Human sperm acrosin as a fertility marker. *J. Androl.*, 8, 20P

Related subjects: pro-acrosin, acrosome reaction, acrosome reaction test, semen analysis — biochemical test of spermatozoa

ACROSOME REACTION

An irreversible event associated with the final phase of capacitation. The acrosome is a membrane-bound organelle that develops from the Golgi apparatus during the spermatid phase of spermatogenesis. It covers the anterior 50–70% of the sperm head. The acrosome reaction involves fusion of the sperm plasma membrane with the outer acrosomal membrane, thereby releasing the acrosomal contents as vesicles and exposing the inner acrosomal membrane. It is an essential part of sperm–zona binding. *In vivo* acrosomal reaction takes place at or near the zona pellucida. Premature acrosome reaction prevents fertilization. Testing of acrosomal reaction can possibly serve as a tool, providing additional information about the fertilizing capacity of a semen sample. See Figures 1, 2 and 3.

1.   Calvo, L., Dennison-Lagos, L., Banks, S.M. and Sherins, R.J. (1994). Characterization and frequency distribution of sperm acrosome reaction among normal and infertile men. *Hum. Reprod.*, 9(10), 1875

2.   Rogers, B.J. and Bentwood, B. (1982). Capacitation, acrosome reaction and fertilization. In Zaneveld, L.J.D. and Chatterton, R.T. (eds.) *Biochemistry of Mammalian Reproduction,* p. 203. (New York: John Wiley & Sons)

3.   Zaneveld, L.J.D., Anderson, R.A., Mack, S.R. and De Jonge, C.J. (1994). Mechanism and control of the human sperm acrosome reaction. *Hum. Reprod.*, 8(12), 2006

Related subjects: capacitation, fertilization, hyperactivation, spermatogenesis, sperm maturation

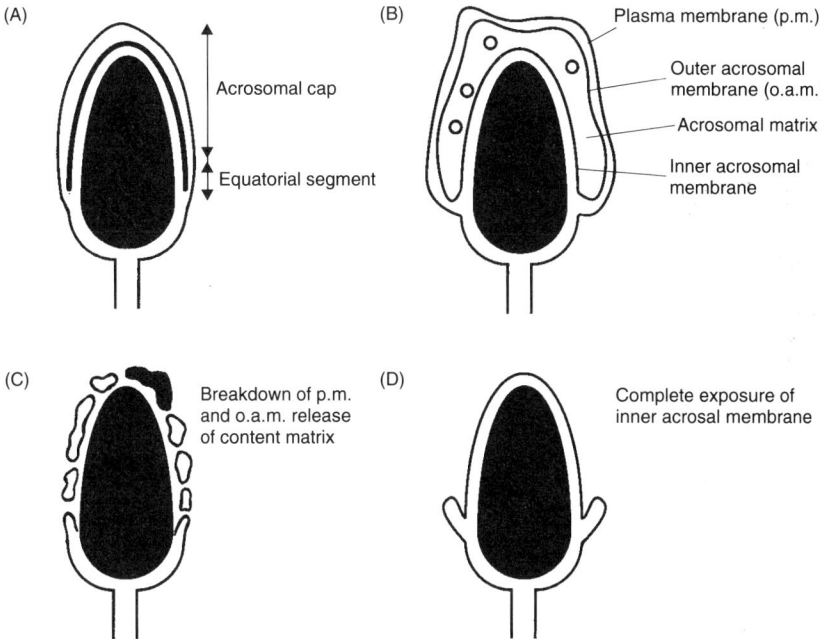

(A)

Acrosomal cap

Equatorial segment

(B)

Plasma membrane (p.m.)

Outer acrosomal membrane (o.a.m.)

Acrosomal matrix

Inner acrosomal membrane

(C)

Breakdown of p.m. and o.a.m. release of content matrix

(D)

Complete exposure of inner acrosal membrane

Figure 1 The acrosome reaction: (A) lifting of plasma membrane; (B) dispersion of outer acrosomal membrane and dissolution of plasma membrane; (C) vesiculation of outer acrosomal membrane; and (D) complete exposure of inner acrosomal membrane

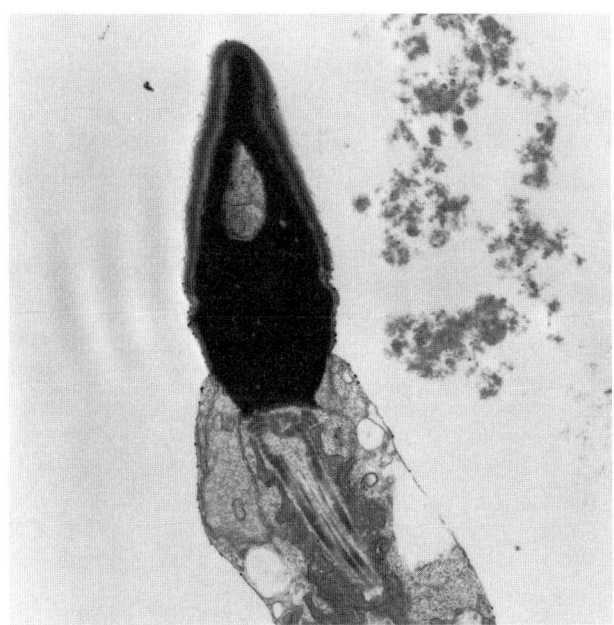

Figure 2 A normal acrosome. Also shown is the equatorial segment and cytoplasmic droplets (see *morphology, abnormal*)

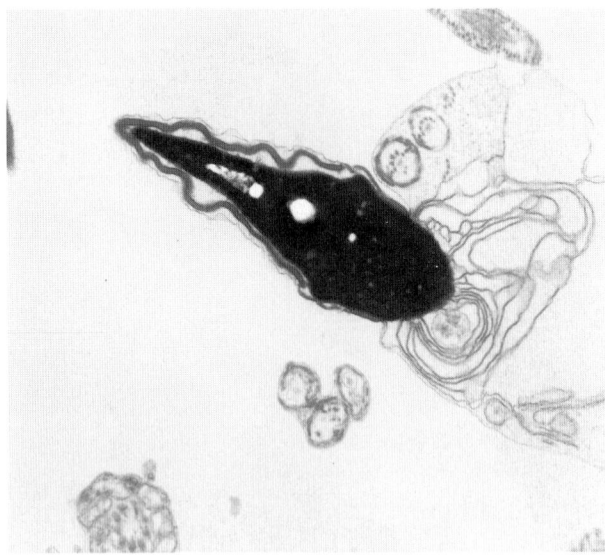

Figure 3   A sperm with an abnormal acrosome. It also shows a slight dag defect (see *morphology, abnormal*)

ACROSOME REACTION, TEST

Laboratory assessment of this process is essential in the case of fertilization failure. As the human acrosomal cap is too small to be visualized directly with phase-contrast microscopy, indirect methods have to be applied:

(1) Staining techniques (e.g. triple stain);

(2) Indirect immunofluorescence with monoclonal antibodies;

(3) Direct immunofluorescence with fluorescein-labelled lectins (these reagents bind to acrosome-associated antigens); and

(4) Electron microscopy (see Figures 4 and 5).

Acrosome-reacted spermatozoa show either no acrosomal labelling or an equatorial band. The predictive value of measuring the acrosome reaction is not known. The development of a bioassay which correlates the fertilizing potential of a capacitated sperm population to the inducibility of the acrosome reaction by ionophore challenge (ARIC) is described.

1.   Calvo, L., Dennison-Lagos, L., Banks, S.M. and Sherins, R.J. (1994). Characterization and frequency distribution of sperm acrosome reaction among normal and infertile men. *Hum. Reprod.*, 9(10), 1875

2.   Carver-Ward, J.A., Jaroudi, K.A., Hollanders, J.M.G., Einspenner, M., Sheth, K.V. and Vemer, H.M. (1996). "Nothing predicts like CD 46" — acrosomal reaction testing with flow cytometry predicts fertilization failure in IVF. *Hum. Reprod.*, in press

3.   Cummins, J.M., Pember, S.M., Jequier, A.M., Yovich, J.L. and Hartmann, P.E. (1991). A test of the human sperm acrosome reaction following ionophore challenge: relationship to fertility and other seminal parameters. *J. Androl.*, 12, 98

Related subjects: acrosome reaction, lectins, microscopy, stains

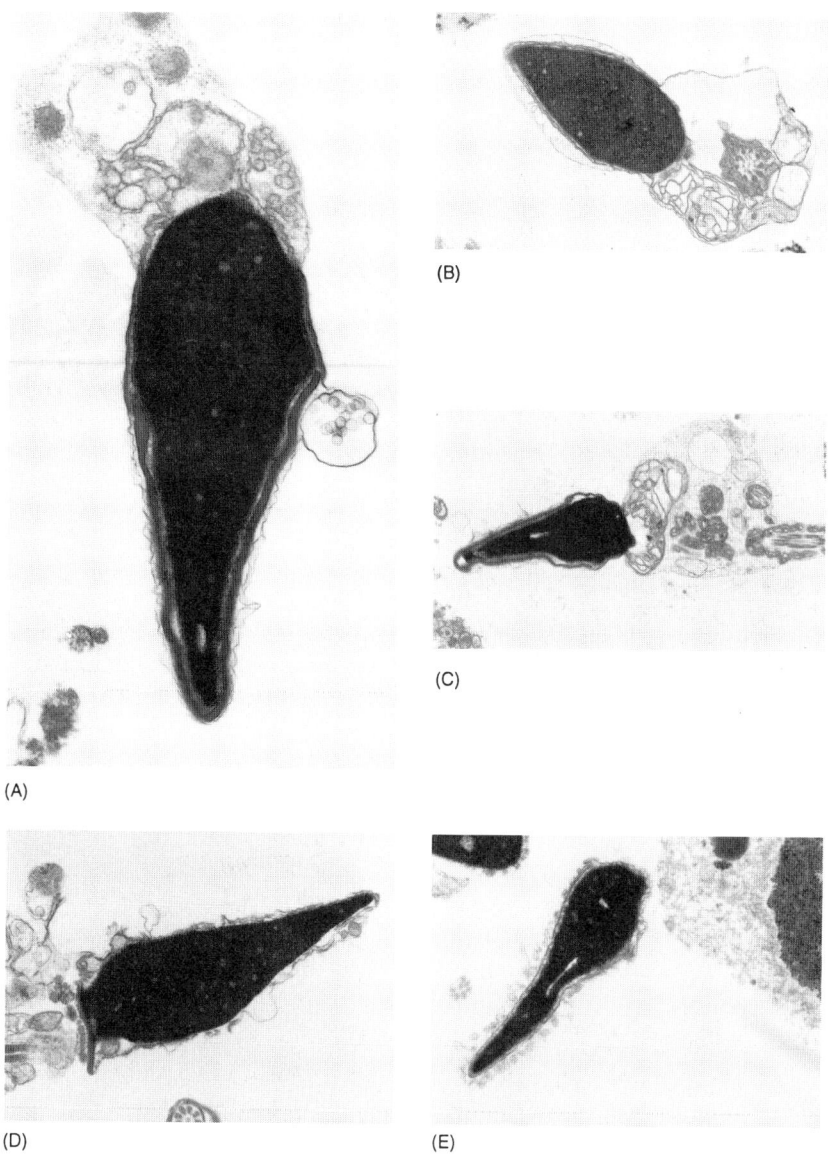

Figure 4 A series of photomicrographs showing the acrosome reaction (AR): (A) the beginning of AR stage I; (B) AR stage I; (C) AR stage I to II (a cytoplasmic droplet is also shown; see *morphology, abnormal*); (D) AR stage II to III; and (E) AR stage III. For stages III to IV see Figure 5

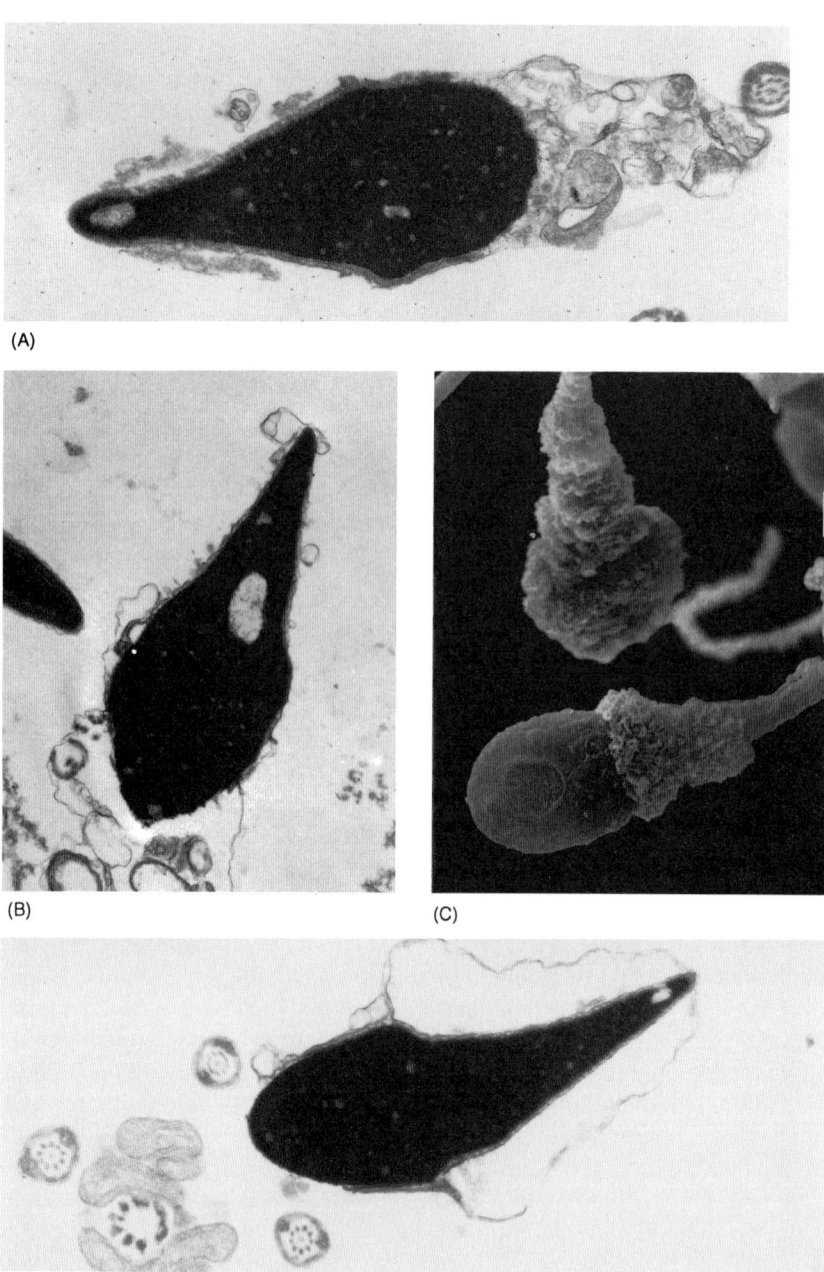

(A)

(B)

(C)

(D)

Figure 5   A series of photomicrographs showing the acrosome reaction (AR): (A) AR stage III to IV; (B and C) AR stage IV; and (D) almost complete stage IV

ACTIVIN

A glycoprotein hormone which is produced in one heterodimer form, activin AB (βA and (βB), and in two homodimer forms, activin A (βA and βA) and activin B (βB and βB). It is secreted by the Leydig cells and possibly by Sertoli cells and stimulates follicle stimulating hormone (FSH) secretion.

1. Veldhuis, J. (1991). The hypothalamic–pituitary–testicular axis. In Yen, S.S.C. and Jaffe, R.B. (eds.) *Reproductive Endocrinology*, 3rd edn. (Philadelphia: W.B. Saunders)

Related subjects: endocrinology, FSH, inhibin, Leydig cell, Sertoli cell

AGGLUTINATION

The process when spermatozoa are bound to each other by antibodies. Normally the spermatozoa are motile, and only a few other cells and debris are seen. In the case of agglutination there is decreased motility and the involvement of other round cells and the amount of debris is minimal. Patterns of agglutination include head-to-head, tail-to-tail and head-to tail agglutination.

Related subjects: antisperm antibodies

AGGREGATION

Clumping of usually dead spermatozoa, mixed with a substantial amount of other cells and debris. Small aggregates are found in almost every semen specimen, large clumps are abnormal.

Related subjects: agglutination, necrozoospermia

AGING

With increasing age there is a significant decrease in sperm motility and increase in sperm density. Other parameters such as morphology, ejaculatory volume and zona-free hamster penetration test show less impressive changes. Semen of men of older age differs from younger men, probably because of significant longer periods of abstinence. Male age is a significant factor contributing to a decreased likelihood in intrauterine insemination treatment. In general, sexual activity decreases with age, possibly due to age-related decline in testosterone levels which goes along with progressively increasing gonadotropin levels. Erectile dysfunction is a major contributory factor: being 2% at age 40, and 50% at age 75. Estradiol, androstenedione and dehydroepiandrosterone levels decrease significantly with age. There is a highly significant age related increase in structural chromosomal abnormalities in spermatozoa: from 2.8% at 20 to 13.6% at 45 years and above. This is reflected in an increased risk for subsequent major birth defects, rising from 0.2/1000 below 30 to around 4/1000 above age 40. Most studies do not show any correlation between paternal age and Down's syndrome. The percentage of X or Y bearing sperm is not related to age.

1. Bordson, B.L. and Leonardo, V.S. (1991). The appropriate upper age limit for semen donors: a review of the genetic effects of paternal age. *Fertil. Steril.*, 56, 397

2. Gerhard, I., Lenhard, K., Eggert-Kruse, W. and Runnebaum, B. (1992). Clinical data which influence semen parameters in infertile men. *Hum. Reprod.*, 7, 830

3. Lian, Z., Zack, M.M. and Erickson, J.J. (1987). Paternal age on the frequency of sperm chromosomal abnormalities in normal men. *Am. J. Hum. Genet.*, 41, 484

4. Mathieu, C., Ecochard, R., Bied, V., Lornage, J. and Czyba, J.C. (1995). Cumulative conception rate following intrauterine artificial insemination with husband's spermatozoa: influence of husband's age. *Hum. Reprod.*, 10(5), 1090

5. Nieschlag, E., Lammers, U. and Freischem, C.W. (1982). Reproductive function in young fathers and grandfathers. *J. Clin. Endocrinol. Metab.*, 55, 676

6. Zenzes, M.T., Reed, T.E. and Nieschlag, E. (1991). Non-poisson distribution of sperm from grandfathers in zona-free hamster ova. *J. Androl.*, 12(1), 71

Related subjects: semen analysis — normal values, sexual dysfunction, chromosomal abnormalities

AGONADISM

Early fetal testicular degeneration between 60 and 69 days after conception is associated with minimal Wolffian development, preserved Mullerian ducts and ambiguous external genitalia. Levels of luteinizing hormone (LH) and follicle stimulating hormone (FSH) are high. The chromosomal structure is 46 XY.

1. Coulam, C.B. (1979). Testicular regression syndrome. *Obstet. Gynecol.*, 53, 44

2. Speroff, L., Glass, R.H. and Kase, N.G. (1993). *Clinical Gynecologic Endocrinology And Infertility*, 5th edn. (Baltimore:Williams and Wilkins)

Related subjects: anorchia, embryology, gonadal dysgenesis, gonadodysgenesis, hypergonadotropic hypogonadism

ALCOHOL

Alcohol (methanol, ethanol, propanol) inhibits the zinc-dependent conversion of vitamin A to bioactive retinol in the testis. Testicular biopsies in alcohol abusers show decreased maturation of the germinal epithelium. Alcohol inhibits testosterone synthesis directly, an action independent of the effect on the liver. In addition, the metabolic clearance rate of testosterone is increased. The hypothalamic–pituitary axis is impaired as well, since low testosterone is not associated with appropriate luteinizing hormone (LH) elevation. Literature generally reports no or moderate alterations in fertility in alcohol users, although postcoital tests show better results in non-alcohol users.

1. Close, C.E., Roberts, P.L. and Berger, R.E. (1990). Cigarettes, alcohol and marijuana are related to pyospermia in infertile men. *J. Urol.*, 144(4), 900–3

2. Feichtinger, W. (1991). Environmental factors and fertility. *Hum. Reprod.*, 6(8), 1170–5

3. Gerhard, I., Lenhard, K., Eggert-Kruse, W. and Runnebaum, B. (1992). Clinical data which influence semen parameters in infertile men. *Hum. Reprod.*, 7, 830–7

4. Kucheria, K., Saxena, R. and Mohan, D. (1985). Semen analysis in alcohol dependence syndrome. *Andrologia*, 17, 558–61

5. Marshburn, P.B., Sloan, C.S. and Hammond, M.G. (1989). Semen quality in association with coffee drinking, cigarette smoking and ethanol consumption. *Fertil. Steril.*, 52, 162–5

Related subjects: history — male infertility, liver disease, nutritional deficiencies, semen analysis — normal values, zinc

AMORPHOUS SPERMATOZOA

A term used for all types of spermatozoa with bizarre forms or with multiple defects, not fitting in any of the main categories of abnormal morphology. Otherwise normal semen analysis may include amorphous spermatozoa.

Related subjects: morphology — abnormal and normal

ANATOMY (Figures 6 and 7)

1. Mortimer, D. (1994). *Practical Laboratory Andrology.* (Oxford: Oxford University Press)

Related subjects: epididymis, prostate, seminal vesicle, testis

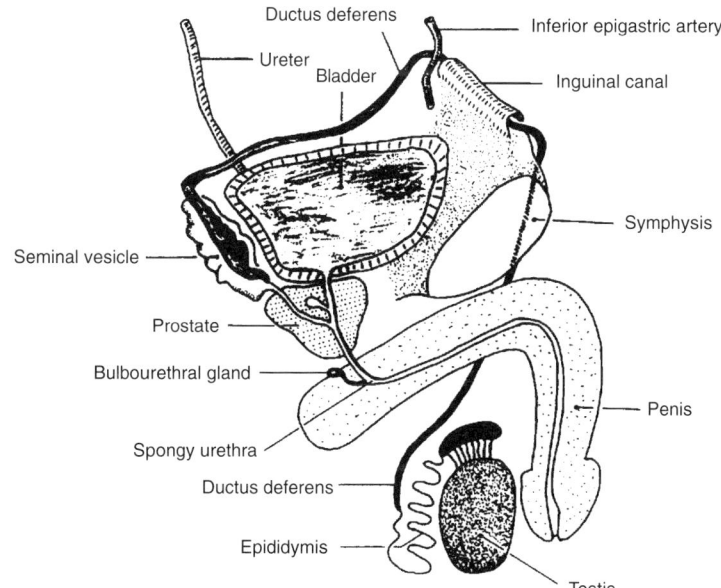

Figure 6 The male reproductive system

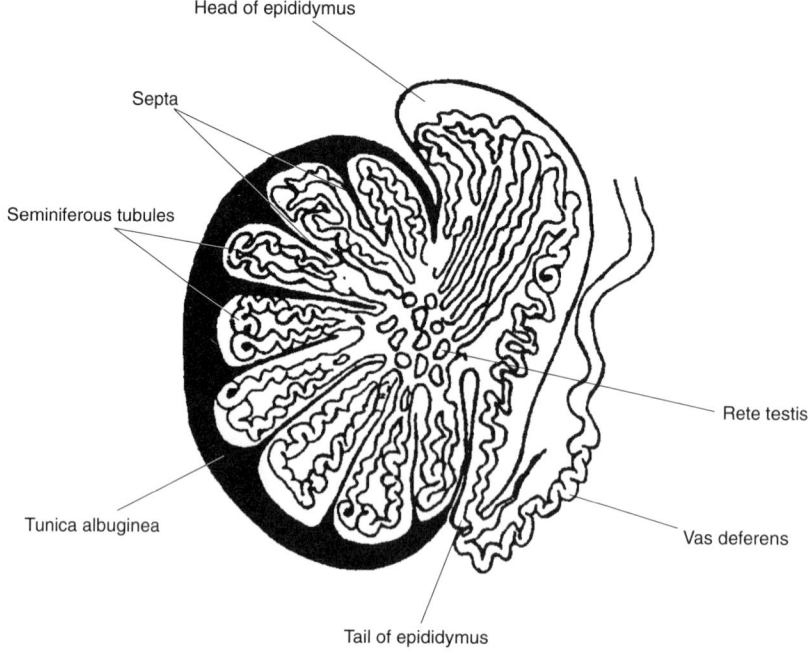

Figure 7 The anatomy of the testis

ANDROGEN BINDING PROTEIN (ABP)

A testis specific protein, synthesized by the Sertoli cells and secreted into the seminiferous tubular fluid. As such, it is a sensitive marker of Sertoli cell function. Synthesis is stimulated by follicle stimulating hormone and by testosterone. Its presence enables the very high intratesticular androgen levels necessary for adequate spermatogenesis. ABP has a strong similarity with testosterone–estradiol binding globulin (TEBG); differences are mainly found in the carbohydrate content.

1. Veldhuis, J. (1991). The hypothalamic–pituitary–testicular axis. In Yen, S.S.C. and Jaffe, R.B. (eds.) *Reproductive Endocrinology*, 3rd edn. (Philadelphia: W.B.Saunders)

Related subjects: endocrinology, Sertoli cell, testosterone–estradiol binding globulin

ANDROGEN INSENSITIVITY SYNDROME

Now used to denote failure of any of the mechanisms involved in the response of target cells to androgens. Since androgens are essential for normal male sexual development, failure of this mechanism to occur will result in anomalous male differentiation. Patients affected with the androgen insensitivity syndrome can present from one extreme side of the spectrum as a phenotypical female to the other end presenting as mildly undervirilized but potentially fertile male. Originally, only one end of the spectrum was described, the testicular feminization syndrome: a form of congenital insensitivity to androgens, caused by an X-linked recessive disorder resulting in 46 XY males with female phenotype, lacking both developed Wolffian and Mullerian ducts. The diagnostic criterion for all forms is the finding of elevated luteinizing hormone and testosterone concentrations in the absence of virilization.

The following categories can be distinguished in individuals with androgen insensitivity:

(1) Absence of androgen receptor binding;

(2) Reduced androgen receptor binding;

(3) Normal binding to abnormal androgen receptor; and

(4) Normal androgen receptor binding but abnormal postreceptor mechanisms.

The phenotypical expression of the syndrome is variable and cannot be related to the type of abnormality in the receptor. This suggests that genetic determinants other than the coding sequence of the androgen receptor will alter the phenotype. Clinically, these patients can be divided into the following groups:

(1) Complete testicular feminization;

(2) Incomplete testicular feminization, Lub's syndrome: assigned sex female but partial Wolffian development, pubic and axillary hair and partial labioscrotal fusion;

(3) Reifenstein's syndrome, males with perineoscrotal hypospadia and bifid or incompletely fused scrotum;

(4) Infertile azoospermic men;

(5) Undervirilized but fertile men.

1. Fauser, B.C.J.M. and Hsueh, A.J.W. (1995). Genetic basis of human reproductive endocrine disorders. *Hum. Reprod.*, 10(4), 826

2. Griffin, J.E. (1992). Androgen resistance — the clinical and molecular spectrum. *N. Engl. J. Med.*, 326, 611

3. McPhaul, M.J., Marcell, M., Zoppi, S., Griffin, J.E. and Wilson, J.D. (1993). Genetic basis of endocrine disease. 4 The spectrum of mutations in the androgen receptor gene that causes androgen resistance. *J. Clin. Endocrinol. Metab.*, 76, 17

4. Morris, J.M. and Mahesh, B.V. (1953). The syndrome of testicular feminization in male pseudohermaphrodites. *Am. J. Obstet. Gynecol.*, 65, 1192

5. Simpson, J.L. (1992). Genetics of sexual differentiation. In Rock, J.A. and Carpenter, S.E. (eds.) *Pediatric and Adolescent Gynecology*, pp. 1–37. (New York: Raven Press)

Related subjects: azoospermia, embryology, genetics, hypergonadotropic hypogonadism, testicular feminization syndrome

ANDROGENS, BIOLOGICAL ACTION

Testosterone has many biological effects in the male. The action of testosterone can be exerted in different ways (Table 1):

(1) Passive diffusion into a tissue and binding to androgen receptor.

(2) Passive diffusion into a tissue, conversion to dihydrotestosterone and binding to androgen receptor.

(3) Passive diffusion into a tissue, aromatization to estradiol and binding to estrogen receptor.

(4) Effect in tissue independent of androgen or estrogen receptor.

Table 1   The action of testosterone

Anabolic	stimulation of body growth, nitrogen retention, muscular development
Maturation of secondary sexual characteristics	accessory sexual organs (penis, aprostate, scrotum, seminal vesicle) growth of larynx and vocal cords male hair growth
Sexual	facilitates libido and potency
Protein synthesis (stimulation or suppression)	liver, kidney, salivary gland
Spermatogenesis	interaction with FSH on Sertoli cell, stimulation of spermatogenesis
Hematopoiesis	stimulation of erythropoietin
Bone	prevention of bone loss
Behavior	assertive, aggressive

1.   Veldhuis, J. (1991). The hypothalamic–pituitary–testicular axis. In Yen, S.S.C. and Jaffe, R.B. (eds.) *Reproductive Endocrinology*, 3rd edn. (Philadelphia: W.B. Saunders)

Related subjects: endocrinology, spermatogenesis, testosterone

ANDROGEN THERAPY

The primary indication is as substitution for sexual dysfunction in hypo-androgenic states, not for treatment of infertility. It has no role in patients with secondary hypogonadism, where fertility is usually achieved by gonadotropin releasing hormone (GnRH) or human menopausal gonadotropin/human chorionic gonadotropin (hMG/hCG). There is no evidence that low-dose androgen therapy is effective in idiopathic oligoasthenospermia. Likewise high-dose testosterone rebound therapy is no longer being used for the same reason. In addition, a small number of patients treated with high-dose androgens have persistently decreased sperm density secondary to the treatment and even cases of permanent azoospermia have been reported.

1. Gerris, J., Comhaire, F., Hellemans, P., Peeters, K. and Schoonjans, F. (1991). Placebo-controlled trial of high-dose mesterolone treatment of idiopathic male infertility. *Fertil. Steril.*, 55, 603–7

2. Pusch, H.H. (1989). Oral treatment of oligozoospermia with testosterone-undecanoate: results of a double-blind-placebo-controlled trial. *Andrologia*, 21, 76

3. Wang, C., Chan, C. and Wong, K. (1983). Comparison of the effectiveness of placebo, clomiphene citrate, mesterolone, pentoxifylline and testosterone rebound therapy for the treatment of idiopathic oligozoospermia. *Fertil. Steril.*, 40, 358

Related subjects: endocrinology, medication — treatment, testosterone rebound therapy

ANEJACULATION

Failure to obtain ejaculation, that is forceful expulsion of the semen from the posterior urethra. Anejaculation can occur as a result of spinal cord injury, retroperitoneal surgery, diabetes mellitus or multiple sclerosis. Treatment nowadays consists of rectal probe electro-ejaculation or penile vibratory stimulation.

Related subjects: azoospermia, electro-ejaculation, paraplegia, retrograde ejaculation, spinal cord injury, vibratory stimulation

ANORCHISM

Late fetal testicular regression after 140 days postconception is associated with male phenotype, but no testes are present. Often called 'the vanishing testis syndrome'. Levels of luteinizing hormone and follicle stimulating hormone are high. The chromosomal sex is 46 XY.

1. Coulam, C.B. (1979). Testicular regression syndrome. *Obstet. Gynecol.*, 53, 44

2. Speroff, L., Glass, R.H. and Kase, N.G. (1993). *Clinical Gynecologic Endocrinology and Infertility*, 5th edn. (Baltimore: Williams and Wilkins)

Related subjects: agonadism, embryology, gonadal dysgenesis, gonadodysgenesis, hypergonadotropic hypogonadism

ANTIBIOTICS, EFFECTS ON SPERMATOGENESIS

The impact of the effects of antibiotics on infertility is perhaps greater than generally assumed. It is well documented that antibiotics like nitrofurantoin and gentamycin can lead to spermatogenic arrest at the spermatocyte level. Although the use of antibiotics has increased greatly in the last decades, direct measurement of the effects on male fertility has many confounding factors. The potentially negative effects of antibiotics on human fertility can be categorized in Table 2.

For the antibiotics as categorized below, so far only animal data are suggestive for possible negative effects on spermatogenesis and/or semen parameters (Table 3).

Table 2 The potential negative effects of antibiotics on male fertility

Antibiotic	Effects in human	Class/comment
Nitrofurantoin	reversible reduction of sperm count — spermatogenic arrest at primary spermatocyte level	nitrofurantoin
Erythromycin	impaired motility during treatment	macrolide
Gentamycin	cessation of meiosis at primary spermatocyte level	aminoglycoside
Neomycin	impaired count and motility	aminoglycoside
Chlortetracyclin	strong negative effect on motility	tetracyclin
Sulfasalazine	impaired count, motility and morphology	sulfa
Co-Trimoxazole	impaired count, motility and morphology	sulfa

Table 3 The potential negative effects of antibiotics on spermatogenesis and sperm parameters

Antibiotic	Animal data	Class/comment
Spiramycin	spermatogenic arrest	macrolide
Lincomycin	decreased motility	macrolide
Tylosin	decreased motility	macrolide
Penicillin G	spermatogenic arrest	
Cephalotin	spermatogenic arrest	penicillin
Ampicillin	decreased fertilizing capacity	penicillin
Dicloxacillin	decreased motility	penicillin
Quinolones	decreased motility	inhibit DNA gyrase — so far, no adverse effects reported

The use of antibiotics in men with an infertility problem, or even without such, should be balanced against the possible negative effects on semen quality of a specific antibiotic. The use of tetracycline with its strong effect on sperm motility, for example, seems to be only justified after thorough evaluation.

1. Schlegel, P.N. Chang, T.S. and Marshall, F.F. (1991). Antibiotics: potential hazards to male infertility. *Fertil. Steril.*, 55(2), 235–42

Related subjects: asthenozoospermia, history male infertility, oligoasthenoteratozoospermia, spermatogenic arrest

ANTI-OXIDANTS

Oxygen radicals are involved in the initiation of peroxidative damage to the sperm plasma membrane. On the other hand, superoxide anions and hydrogen peroxide also participate in the induction of biological key events such as hyperactivated motility and acrosome reaction. Thus human spermatozoa appear to use reactive oxygen species for different physiological purposes. Anti-oxidants like vitamin C, vitamin E, taurine, hypotaurine and glutathione can possibly protect against negative effects on sperm quality and against oxidative DNA damage, especially under circumstances of oxidative stress such as is the case in laboratory handling of semen samples with poor quality spermatozoa or leukocytes. The negative effects of smoking may also be attributed to oxidative stress, especially in heavy smokers.

1. Aitken, J. and Fisher, H. (1994). Reactive oxygen species generation and human spermatozoa: the balance of benefit and risk. *Bioessays*, 16(4), 259–67

2. Guerin, P., Guillaud, J. and Menezo, Y. (1995). Hypotaurine in spermatozoa and genital secretions and its production by oviduct epithelial cells *in vitro. Hum. Reprod.*, 10(4), 866

3. Lenzi, A., Culasso, F. and Gandini, L. (1993). Placebo-controlled, double-blind, cross-over trial of glutathione therapy in male infertility. *Hum. Reprod.*, 8, 1657

4. Moilanen, J., Hovatta, O. and Lindroth, L. (1993). Vitamin E levels in seminal plasma can be elevated by oral administration of vitamin E in infertile men. *Int. J. Androl.*, 16(2), 165–6

Related subjects: cigarette smoking, leukocytospermia, medication — treatment, oxygen — reactive species, sperm preparation techniques

ANTISPERM ANTIBODIES

Antisperm antibodies can be found in the serum of male or female, in seminal plasma, on the surface of the spermatozoon and in cervical mucus. The antibodies can be circulating in the serum and enter the seminal plasma or cervical mucus through transudation, or can be produced locally in the male sexual accessory glands or in the cervix. The mechanisms through which antisperm antibodies can interfere with fertility are decreased sperm motility, an increased number of of non-viable sperm, impaired sperm–mucus penetration, alterations in capacitation and acrosomal reaction and interference with sperm–oocyte interaction. The incidence of positive antisperm antibodies is higher in subfertile populations. Two types of sperm antibodies can be distinguished: immobilizing (cell toxic) and agglutinating antibodies. In serum mainly IgG and IgM are found, while IgA is present locally in the genital tract. IgA affects fertilization *in vitro* when present on the sperm head; IgM has to be localized on the head and the tail to cause this drop in fertilization. Testing for antibodies is indicated in patients with spontaneous agglutination in the ejaculate, in cases of poor motility or a low number of live spermatozoa, in those with poor sperm–mucus interaction (especially when sperm shaking is present), in unexplained infertility and before vasectomy reversal. There are numerous tests for antisperm antibodies, but only a few are valid in terms of sensitivity, specificity and reproducibility. Only the mixed antiglobulin reaction test (MAR) and the immunobead test (IBT) are of value for routine clinical purpose (see Table 4).

Table 4 The tests for antisperm antibodies in men

Test	Mechanism	Comment
Mixed antiglobulin reaction (MAR)	sperm agglutinates in the presence of IgG and IgA antiserum to (sheep) red blood cells it is a modified Coombs' test	is highly specific for IgG, less for IgA can only be used on motile sperm no sperm preparation needed, therefore fast necessary volume only 0.01 ml has to be done within 60 minutes after ejaculation
Immunobead test (IBT)	antihuman antibodies bound to micronsize polyacrylamide spheres complex with antisperm antibodies	for IgG, IgA, IgM can only be used on motile sperm direct test: identifies sperm membrane-bound antibodies indirect test identifies antisperm antibodies in reproductive tract secretions washing of sperm needed – more time-consuming necessary volume 0.2–2.0 ml

1. Adeghe, J.H.A. (1992). Male subfertility due to sperm antibodies: a clinical overview. *Obstet. Gynecol. Surv.*, **48**, 1

2. Bronson, R.A. and Fusi, F.M. (1995). The reproductive immunology of fertilization failure. *Assist. Reprod. Rev.*, **5**(1), 14

3. Clarke, G.N. (1988). Sperm antibodies and human fertilization. *Am. J. Reprod. Immunol. Microbiol.*, **17**, 65

4. Marshburn, P.B. (1994). The role of antisperm antibodies in infertility. *Fertil. Steril.*, 61(5), 799–811

5. Siegel, M.S. (1993). The male fertility investigation and the role of the andrology laboratory. *J. Reprod. Med.*, 38(5), 317

6. Yeh, W.R., Acosta, A.A., Seltman, H.J. and Doncel, G. (1995). Impact of immunoglobulin isotype and sperm surface location of antisperm antibodies on fertilization *in vitro* in the human. *Fertil. Steril.*, 63(6), 1287

Related subjects: agglutination, asthenozoospermia, blood–testis barrier, cryptorchidism, medication — treatment, oligoasthenoteratozoospermia, sperm function test, vasectomy reversal

ANTISPERM ANTIBODIES, TREATMENT

Treatment should only be considered for patients in whom more than 50% of spermatozoa are agglutinated by antibodies, since postcoital tests in patients with lower numbers of agglutinated spermatozoa are normal. The following treatments for antisperm antibodies have been advocated.

(1) Condom therapy has not been shown to decrease antisperm antibody titers or increase the pregnancy rates.

(2) Sperm washing: rapid repeated washings of the ejaculate may remove free antibodies in seminal plasma but not those bound to the sperm surface. Variable success rates are reported.

(3) Some attempts have been made to separate the antibody-free spermatozoa employing Sephadex. On the other hand, literature reports the use of protease addition to the culture medium in an attempt to disagglutinate the spermatozoa.

(4) Immunosuppression:

  (a) Corticosteroids can decrease antibody production and antibody–antigen binding. In the literature there is no agreement on dosage, dosage intervals or duration of treatment. Many reports include uncontrolled variables. Only two studies are placebo and/or double-blind crossover controlled. The results are contradictory possibly due to differences in administration of the drug continuous versus cyclic and duration of treatment. High-dose regimens have been abandonded because of serious side-effects.

  (b) Cyclosporin: only a limited number of reports are available, none are placebo controlled.

(5) Intrauterine insemination: so far, no well controlled study has been reported and success rates are low. IUI seems to have a limited role for isolated immunologic problems. However, one study reports that if cyclical intermediate corticosteroid therapy is combined with IUI, pregnancy rates increase significantly.

(6) Assisted reproductive techniques (ART): although successful reports about ART for immunological male infertility are available, success rates seem to be lower than in non-immunological male infertility. Again, most reports do not include a control group.

1. Haas, G.G. Jr. (1991). Male infertility and immunity. In Lipshultz, L.I. and Howards, S.S. (eds.) *Infertility in the Male*, 2nd edn. (St Louis: Mosby-Year Book)

2. Haas, G.G. Jr, D'Cruz, O.J. and Denum, B.M. (1988). Effect of repeated washing on spermbound immunoglobulin-G. *J. Androl.*, 9, 190

3. Haas, G.G. Jr and Manganiello, P. (1987). A double-blind, placebo-controlled study of the use of methylprednisolone in infertile men with sperm-bound immunoglobulins. *Fertil. Steril.*, 47, 295

4. Hendry, W.F., Hughes, L. and Scammell, G. (1990). Comparison of prednisolone and placebo in subfertile men with antibodies to spermatozoa. *Lancet*, 335–85

5. Isojima, Li T.S. and Ashitaka, Y. (1968). Immunologic analysis of sperm mobilizing factor found in sera of women with unexplained infertility. *Am. J. Obstet.Gynecol.*, 101, 677

6. Pattinson, H.A., Mortimer, D. and Taylor, P.J. (1990). Treatment of spermagglutination with proteolytic enzymes II. Sperm function after enzymatic disagglutination. *Hum. Reprod.*, 5, 174

7. Robinson, J.N., Forman, R.G., Nicholson, S.C., Maciocia, L.R. and Barlow, D.H. (1995). A comparison of intra-uterine insemination in superovulated cycles to intercourse in couples where the male is receiving steroids for the treatment of autoimmune infertility. *Fertil. Steril.*, 63(6), 1260

Related subjects: antisperm antibodies, corticosteroids, Hendry schedule, insemination, medication — treatment, medication — negative effects, sperm preparation

ASPERMIA

Absence of seminal fluid after ejaculation.

Related subjects: azoospermia, retrograde ejaculation

ASSISTED REPRODUCTION

Assisted reproduction means any medical technique interfering with one or more of the mechanisms or barriers that have to be completed before successful fertilization can occur (Table 5).

Identification of a male factor in infertility patients and identifying those for assisted reproduction is handicapped by the lack of uniformity in criteria used. Unlike the clinical male factor which uses pregnancy as a measurable end-point, the end-point for male factor in assisted reproduction is usually the fertilization rate. Depending on the basic semen parameters, the results of sperm function tests and semen preparation, it has to be decided if (and if so which form of) assisted reproductive technique should be applied in case of male factor infertility. Although in particular the successful

Table 5 Comparison of assisted reproductive techniques

		Technique							
		IUI	DIPI	GIFT	ZIFT	IVF/ET	ZD-PZD	SUZI	ICSI
Bypass cervical mucus		yes	yes	yes	yes	yes	—	—	—
Selection of sperm on motility and morphology	sperm preparation	yes	yes	yes	yes	yes	yes	yes	yes
Increase number of mature oocytes	ovarian hyperstimulation	yes/no	yes	yes	yes	yes	—	—	—
Timing of ovulation	hCG	yes/no	yes	yes	yes	yes	—	—	—
Bypass pick-up mechanism	collection of oocytes	no	no	yes	yes	yes	—	—	—
Bypass tubal passage sperm		no	yes	yes	yes	yes	—	—	—
Bypass acrosomal reaction		no	no	no	no	no	no	no	yes
Bypass zona binding		no	no	no	no	no	no	yes	yes
Bypass zona penetration		no	no	no	no	no	no	yes	yes
Bypass fusion with oolemma		no	no	no	no	no	no	no	yes
Selection of oocytes on fertilization		no	no	no	yes	no	—	—	—
Selection of embryos on quality		no	no	no	no	yes	—	—	—
Bypass tubal passage fertilized oocyte		no	no	no	no	yes	—	—	—

IUI = intrauterine insemination, DIPI = direct intraperitoneal insemination, GIFT = gamete intrafallopian transfer, ZIFT = zygote intrafallopian transfer, IVF/ET = *in vitro* fertilization/embryo transfer, ZD-PZD = zona drilling – partial zona dissection, SUZI = subzonal insemination, ICSI = intracytoplasmic sperm injection

introduction of intracytoplasmic sperm injection (ICSI) has brought about major changes in the treatment strategies for men with poor semen quality, as a general guideline the following is still valid:

(1) Intrauterine insemination needs a minimum of at least 1.5 million motile spermatozoa after preparation.

(2) *In vitro* fertilization (IVF) requires about 50 000 motile sperm per inseminated oocyte.

(3) Indications for ICSI are not clearly defined yet. Usually repeated fertilization failure in previous IVF, sperm parameters that primarily do not meet criteria for IVF or results of sperm function tests indicating that acrosome reaction, zona binding or zona penetration potential are severely impaired are considered to be valid indications for ICSI.

1. Acosta, A.A., Swanson, R.J., Ackermann, S.B., Kruger, T.F.,van Zyl, J.A. and Menkveld, R. (1990). *Human Spermatozoa in Assisted Reproduction.* (Baltimore: Williams and Wilkins)

2. Irriani, F.M. and Coddington, C.C. (1992). Male factor infertility and assisted reproductive technologies. *Curr. Opin. Obstet. Gynecol.*, 4, 712

3. Oehninger, S., Stecker, J.F. and Acosta, A.A. (1992). Male infertility: the impact of assisted reproductive technologies. *Curr. Opin. Obstet. Gynecol.*, 4, 185

Related subjects: ICSI, insemination, IVF, micromanipulation, oligoasthenoteratozoospermia, sperm function test

ASTHENOZOOSPERMIA

Less than 50% of sperm are progressively motile (World Health Organization). All other semen parameters are normal. As a single abnormality isolated asthenozoospermia has a frequency of 20%. Etiology includes the factors shown in Table 6.

Table 6   The etiology of asthenozoospermia

Cause	Comment
Developmental	abnormalities before spermiation including chromosomal aberrations
Morphological	structural abnormalities of tail, mid-piece or head (Kartagener's, short-tail syndrome)
Post-spermiation	pathological circumstances: varicocele, infections, toxins, hematospermia, contamination with urine, immobilizing antibodies
Artifacts	inadequate collection, long interval between ejaculation and examination, or inadequate handling in the laboratory

1. Menkveld, R. and Kruger, T.F. (1990). Basic semen analysis. In Acosta, A.A. (ed.) *Human Spermatozoa in Assisted Reproduction.* (Baltimore: Williams and Wilkins)

2. Mundy, A.J., Ryder, T.A. and Edmonds, D.K. (1995). Asthenozoospermia and the human sperm mid-piece. *Hum. Reprod.*, 10(1), 116

3. World Health Organization (1992). *Laboratory Manual for the Examination of Human Semen and Semen Cervical Mucus Interaction.* (Geneva: World Health Organization)

Related subjects: antisperm antibodies, chromosomal abnormalities, hematospermia, morphology — abnormal, motility, semen analysis — collection of sample, seminal plasma motility inhibitor, teratozoospermia, varicocele

AZOOSPERMIA

Absence of spermatozoa in the seminal fluid. Etiologically, the following categories can be distinguished (Table 7).

Table 7 The etiology of azoospermia

Pre-testicular	disorders of hypothalamic–pituitary axis	gonadotropin deficiency syndromes (e.g. Kallmann's) prolactinoma androgen insensitivity syndromes congenital adrenal hyperplasia
Testicular	impaired spermatogenesis	genetic: XXY, trisomy 21, translocation developmental: cryptorchidism, anorchism, germ cell aplasia, Sertoli cell-only environment: heat, drugs, radiation post-mumps autoimmune
Post-testicular	abnormalities epididymis and ejaculatory ducts sexual dysfunction	congenital: absence vas deferens stenosis post-infectious obstruction post-surgical obstruction retrograde ejaculation

Related subjects: azoospermia — flowsheet, androgen insensitivity, chromosomal abnormalities, congenital adrenal hyperplasia, congenital absence vas deferens, cryptorchidism, Down's Syndrome, hypergonadotropic hypogonadism, hypogonadotropic hypogonadism, Kartagener's syndrome, mumps, obstruction, radiation, retrograde ejaculation, sexual dysfunction

AZOOSPERMIA FACTOR (AZF)

This is a gene controlling spermatogenesis. It is located within interval 6 of the human Y chromosome's long arm. Loss of the most distal part is associated with severe spermatogenic impairment. The testis shows absent or severely reduced germ cell development.

1. Kun Ma., Inglis, J.D., Sharkey, A., Bickmore, W.A., Hill, R.E., Prosser, E.J., Speed, R.M., Thomson, E.J., Jobling M., Taylor K., Wolfe J., Cooke, H.J., Hargreave, T.B. and

Chandley, A.C. (1993). A Y chromosome gene family with RNA binding protein homology: candidates for the azoospermia factor AZF controlling human spermatogenesis. *Cell,* 75, 1287–95

2. Simpson, E., Chandler, P., Goulmy, E., Kun Ma., Hargreave, T.B. and Chandley, A.C. (1993). Loss of the "azoospermia factor" on Yq in man is not associated with loss of HYA. *Hum. Mol. Genet.*, 2(4), 469–71

Related subjects: embryology, spermatogenesis , testis determining factor, Y chromosome

AZOOSPERMIA, FLOWSHEET DIAGNOSIS AND MANAGEMENT

As a guideline for the workup of azoospermia the algorithm shown in Figure 8 is suggested.

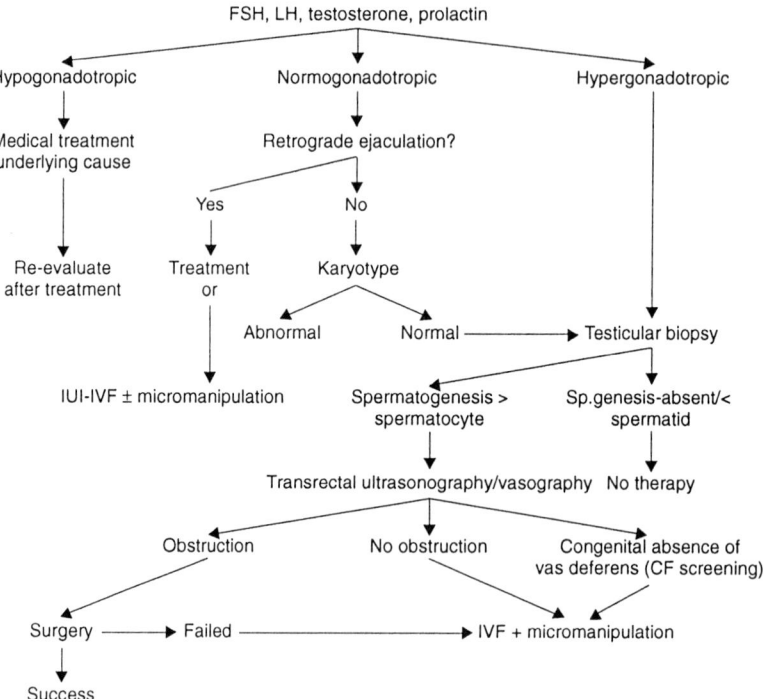

Figure 8   The management of azoospermia. FSH = follicle stimulating hormone; LH = luteinizing hormone; IUI = intrauterine insemination; IVF = *in vitro* fertilization; CF = cystic fibrosis

Related subjects: azoospermia, hypogonadotropic hypogonadism, hypergonadotropic hypogonadism, obstruction, retrograde ejaculation, testicular biopsy, sperm collection techniques

B*b*

BACTERIAL INFECTION

The majority of men with increased number of bacteria and/or leukocytes are asymptomatic. The effect on semen parameters is controversial, with some reports suggesting no effect while others showing reduced semen volume, sperm count, motility and normal morphology. These effects are thought to be secondary to oxidative stress and secretion of cytotoxic cytokines. The criteria for diagnosis are controversial, but normal ejaculate should not contain more than 5×10^6 round cells/ml and 1×10^6 leukocytes/ml; when these values are exceeded semen culture is indicated.

1. Bar-Chama, N., Goluboff, E. and Fisch, H. (1994). Infection and pyospermia in male infertility. Is it really a problem? [review]. *Urol. Clin. N. Am.*, **21**, 469

2. World Health Organization (1992). *Laboratory Manual for the Examination of Human Semen and Semen Cervical Mucus Interaction.* (Geneva: World Health Organization)

Related subjects: culture — semen, leukocytospermia, prostatitis, sexually transmitted diseases

BLOOD–TESTIS BARRIER

The blood–testis barrier is formed by tight junctional complexes between the Sertoli cells, separating the basal component from the luminal compartment. Spermatogonia and young spermatocytes are outside the barrier in the basal part, while mature spermatocytes and spermatids are in the adluminal compartment. The barrier is not formed before puberty. It regulates the access of hormones and metabolites to the germinal cells. It selectively limits the entry of interstitial fluid into the seminiferous tubules and limits the exit of spermatozoa and related antigenic substances. Disruption of this border by injury or infection of the testis or epididymis or by vasectomy invokes a potent antisperm antibody response because of the penetration of sperm antigen into blood and lymph vessels.

1. Setchell, B.P., Maddocks, S. and Brooks, D.E. (1994). Anatomy, vasculature, innervation and fluids of the male genital tract. In Knobil, E. and Neill, J.D. (eds.) *Physiology of Reproduction*, 2nd edn, pp. 1063–175. (New York: Raven Press)

Related subjects: anatomy, antisperm antibodies, Sertoli cell

BROMOCRIPTINE

This is a dopamine agonist. Treatment with bromocriptine increases sperm density and motility and improves sexual dysfunction if present in patients with hyperprolactinemia. The usual dose is 2.5–7.5 mg/day. There is no role for bromocriptine in treatment of idiopathic oligozoospermia in the absence of elevated serum prolactin level.

1. James, H., Gilbaugh III, L.I. and Lipshultz (1994). Non-surgical treatment of male infertility. *Urol. Clin. N. Am.*, 21(3), 541

2. O'Donovan, P.A., Vandekerckhove, P., Lilford, R.J. and Hughes, E. (1993). Treatment of male infertility: is it effective? Review and meta-analyses of published randomized controlled trials. *Hum. Reprod.*, 8, 1209–22

Related subjects: hyperprolactinemia, medication — treatment, microadenoma

Cc

CANDIDIASIS

Candida albicans is a normal inhabitant of the lower gastrointestinal tract. In males retained heat and moisture under the foreskin can cause candidal balanitis. It frequently follows intercourse with an affected partner. Partners should be treated at the same time. Diabetes mellitus should be excluded in men with (recurrent) candidal balanitis. Semen parameters are not impaired.

1. Vohra, S. and Badlani, G. (1992). Balanitis and balanoposthitis. In Mellinger, B.C. and Smith, A.D. (eds.) Sexually transmitted diseases. *Urol. Clin. N. Am.*, 19(1)

Related subjects: diabetes mellitus, sexually transmitted diseases

CAPACITATION

This may be described as a hormone-dependent, estrogen-stimulated event which usually occurs when spermatozoa enter the female reproductive tract and must occur before a spermatozoon is capable of fertilizing a mature oocyte. Capacitation can be considered to be the final step in the maturation process of spermatozoa. Capacitation centers around destabilization of the sperm membrane, thereby increasing permeability and membrane fluidity. This is promoted by:

(1) Separation of the spermatozoon from the seminal plasma, as occurs during passage through the cervical canal (seminal plasma contains several decapacitation factors).

(2) Efflux of cholesterol and influx of unsaturated fatty acids.

(3) Influx of calcium, sodium, potassium, glucose and oxygen, which trigger capacitation and the acrosome reaction.

All stages of capacitation are reversible; the acrosome reaction is not. Although capacitation is considered to be a preparational step for hyperactivation, it is not really clear why capacitation has to preceed the acrosome reaction. Prematurity of the acrosome reaction or hyperactivation prevents sperm–zona binding. All stages of the capacitation process may be induced and observed under *in vitro* conditions.

1. Fraser, L.R. (1992). Requirements for successful mammalian sperm capacitation and fertilzation. *Arch. Pathol. Lab. Med.*, 116(4), 345–50

2. Rogers, B.J. and Bentwood, B. (1982). Capacitation, acrosome reaction and fertilization.

In Zaneveld, L.J.D. and Chatterton, R.T. (eds.) *Biochemistry of Mammalian Reproduction.* (New York: John Wiley & Sons)

Related subjects: acrosome reaction, culture media, fertilization, hyperactivation, sperm maturation, sperm preparation, taurine, zona-free hamster egg penetration test

CARNITINE

Seminal carnitine is a representative parameter for epididymal function, especially the cauda epididymis. It is significantly lower in azoospermic and oligospermic men. In normospermic men motility is better in those with high carnitine levels than in those with low carnitine levels.

1. Micic, S.R., Lalic, N.D. and Dotlic, R.D. (1994). Seminal carnitine and glucosidase in oligospermic and azoospermic men. *J. Androl.*, 15, 77S

Related subjects: semen analysis, biochemical test seminal plasma

CHEMOTHERAPY, EFFECTS ON SPERMATOGENESIS

The occurrence of azoospermia depends on dose, duration, number and type of drugs used. In addition, reversibility is dependent on total dose, duration, type of drug and elapsed time since cessation of therapy: recovery of spermatogenesis is not predictable and can be expected up to 5 years after the end of treatment. Often fertility is already reduced before the start of treatment: 20–40% of Hodgkin patients have oligozoospermia, up to 70% asthenozoospermia. One-half of the patients with germinal cell tumors have an initially low sperm count. Pretreatment cryopreservation of semen has to be included in the management plan. Spermatozoa collected during or after chemotherapy bear considerable risk for genetic damage. Since the success rate of frozen/thawed spermatozoa has greatly improved since the introduction of *in vitro* fertilization (IVF) and micromanipulation procedures, nowadays almost any semen specimen can be cryopreserved regardless of the quality. Protection of spermatogenesis against cytotoxicity by androgen deprivation through suppression with luteinizing hormone-releasing hormone (LHRH) analogue or combinations of androgens and progestogens has been observed in animals but not in humans. The incidence of birth defects and childhood cancer in the offspring of surviving men are the same as found in the general population. The following cytostatics are known to have an adverse effect on spermatogenesis: busulfan, chlorambucil, cyclophosphamide, cytarabine, corticosteroids, doxorubicine (Adriamycin), methotrexate, nitrogen mustard, procarbazine, vinblastine, vincristine. The combinations are:

ABVD: doxorubicin/bleomycin/vinblastine/dacarbazine
CDDP: vinblastine/bleomycin/cisplatin
MOPP: nitrogen mustard/vincristine/prednisolone/procarbazine
MVPP: nitrogen mustard/vinblastine/prednisolone/procarbazine

1. Berthelsen, J.G. and Skakkebaek, N.S. (1983). Gonadal fuction in men with testis cancer. *Fertil. Steril.*, 39(1), 68

2. Byrne, J. (1990). Fertility and pregnancy after malignancy. *Semin. Perinatol.*, 14, 423

3. Dukes, M.N.G. (ed.) (1988). *Meyler's Side Effects of Drugs. An Encyclopedia of Adverse Reactions and Interactions.* (Amsterdam: Elsevier)

4. Glantz, J.C. (1994). Reproductive toxicology of alkylating agents. *Obstet. Gynecol. Surv.*, 49(10), 709

5. Hendry, W.F., Stedronska, J. and Jones, C.R. (1983). Semen analysis in testicular cancer and Hodgkin's disease: pre- and posttreatment findings and implications for for cryopreservation. *Br. J. Urol.*, 55, 769

6. Meistrich, M.L. (1993). Potential genetic risks of using semen collected during chemotherapy. *Hum. Reprod.*, 8(1), 8

7. Morris, I.D. (1993). Protection agianst cytotoxic induced testis damage — experimental approaches. *Eur. Urol.*, 23(1), 143

8. Neumann, F. (1984). Effects of drugs and chemicals on spermatogenesis. *Arch. Toxicol. Suppl.*, 7, 109

9. Oates, R.D. and Lipshultz, L.I. (1989). Fertility and testicular function in patients after radiotherapy and chemotherapy. In Lytton, B. (ed.) *Advances in Urology*, Vol.2, p. 55. (Chicago: Mosby-Year Book)

10. Parvinen, M., Lahdetie, J. and Parvinen, L.-M. (1984). Toxic and mutagenic influences on spermatogenesis. *Arch. Toxicol. Suppl.*, 7, 147

Related subjects: azoospermia, chromosomal abnormalities — sperm cells, cryopreservation, germ cell mutagens, hypergonadotropic hypogonadism, spermatogenic arrest, testicular biopsy — histopathology

CHLAMYDIA TRACHOMATIS

This is an obligatory intracellular bacterium and one of the main causes of non-specific urethritis and epididymitis (30–40%). It is also found in 15–35% of men with gonococcal infection. As many as 20% of men with chlamydial urethritis are asymptomatic. The major complication is epididymitis, presenting as an acute tender testicular swelling. It is the most common cause of epididymitis in males under 40 years of age. Infection with *Chlamydia* may depress semen parameters, possibly because of immune-related infertility. It has been shown that *Chlamydia* infection activates T cells, thus possibly leading to antisperm antibody formation. Doxycycline (100 mg b.i.d. for 7–10 days), erythromycin (500 mg q.i.d. for 7–10 days) or quinolones are the antibiotic treatment of choice.

1. Zenilman, J.M. (1992). Update on bacterial sexually transmitted disease. In Mellinger, B.C. and Smith, A.D. (eds.) *Urol. Clin. N. Am.*, 19(1), 25

2. Autoimmunity to spermatozoa, asymptomatic *Chlamydia trachomatis* genital tract infection and T lymphocytes in seminal fluid from the male partners of couples with unexplained infertility. *Hum. Reprod.*, 10(5), 1070

Related subjects: antisperm antibodies, gonococcal infection, sexually transmitted diseases

CHROMOSOMAL ABNORMALITIES, SOMATIC CELLS

It is estimated that around 12% of men with azoospermia and 7% with severe oligozoospermia have abnormal somatic cell karyotyping: mainly XXY or translocations.

1. De Braekeleer, M. and Dao, T.N. (1991). Cytogenetic studies in male infertility: a review. *Hum. Reprod.*, 6(2), 245

Related subjects: azoospermia, hypergonadotropic hypogonadism

CHROMOSOMAL ABNORMALITIES, SPERM CELLS

The significance of chromosomal anomalies in sperm cells is controversial. Some can be found in fertile men. Normal human sperm cells are prone to *de novo* structural abnormalities (7.5%). The most common are chromosome breaks and chromosome fragments. Usually chromosomes have been examined after fusion with zona-free hamster eggs, but more recently fluorescent *in-situ* hybridization (FISH) is being employed with interphase sperm nuclei. The problem of losing normal sperm morphology and the sperm tails after DNA decondensation necessary for FISH now seems to be overcome by recent modifications of the procedure.

Storage of spermatozoa after *in vitro* incubation may alter the number of structural abnormalities up to threefold. Aneuploidy and sex ratio are not affected by the procedure. Cryopreservation of spermatozoa does not affect any of the variables mentioned.

1. Estop, A.M., Cieply, K., Vankirk, V., Munne, S. and Garver, K. (1991). Cytogenetic studies in human sperm. *Hum. Genet.*, 87, 447
2. Martin, R.H., Chernos, J.E. and Rademaker, A.W. (1991). Effect of cryopreservation on the frequency of chromosomal abnormalities and sex ratio in human sperm. *Mol. Reprod. Dev.*, 30(2), 159
3. Martin, R.H. (1993). Detection of genetic damage in human sperm. *Reprod. Toxicol.*, 7(Suppl. 1), 47
4. Martini, E., Speel, E.J.M., Geraedts, J.P.M., Ramaekers, F.C.S. and Hopman, A.H.N. (1995). Application of different *in situ* hybridization detection methods for human sperm analysis. *Hum. Reprod.*, 10(4), 855
5. Munne, S. and Estop, A.M. (1993). Chromosome analysis of human spermatozoa stored *in vitro*. *Hum. Reprod.*, 8(4), 581

Related subjects: cryopreservation, chemotherapy

CIGARETTE SMOKING

Most reports in the literature show a dose-related effect of smoking on semen volume and motility. Figures relating to morphology and sperm count are conflicting. Smokers have elevated levels of estradiol, testosterone, dihydrotestosterone and lower levels of prolactin when compared to non-smokers. Possible etiological factors might be a decrease in the amount of seminal zinc and an increase in seminal cadmium in heavy smokers. In addition, cigarette smokers show an increased number of seminal fluid leukocytes. The negative effect of smoking on sperm parameters may possibly be averted by high-dose ascorbic acid, protecting the sperm cells against endogenous oxidative DNA damage. There is no evidence that maternal smoking during pregnancy has significant effects on semen characteristics, hormone levels or fertility in male offspring.

1. Close, C.E., Roberts, P.L. and Berger, R.E. (1990). Cigarettes, alcohol and marijuana are related to pyospermia in infertile men. *J. Urol.*, 144(4), 900

2. Dawson, E.B., Harris, W.A., Teter, M.C. and Powell, L.C. (1992). Effect of ascorbic acid supplementation on the sperm quality of smokers. *Fertil. Steril.*, 58(5), 1034

3. Gerhard, I., Lenhard, K., Eggert-Kruse, W. and Runnebaum, B. (1992). Clinical data which influence semen parameters in infertile men. *Hum. Reprod.*, 7, 830

4. Marshburn, P.B., Sloan, C.S. and Hammond, M.G. (1989). Semen quality in association with coffee drinking, cigarette smoking and ethanol consumption. *Fertil. Steril.*, 52, 162

5. Parazzini, F., Marchini, M., Tozzi, L., Mezzopane, R. and Fedele, L. (1993). Risk factors for unexplained dyspermia in infertile men: a case–control study. *Arch. Androl.*, 31(2), 105

6. Ratcliffe, J.M., Gladen, B.C., Wilcox, A.J. and Herbst, A.L. (1992). Does early exposure to maternal smoking affect future in adult males? *Reprod. Toxicol.*, 6(4), 297

Related subjects: antioxidants, history — male infertility, leucocytopspermia, medication — treatment, occupational hazards, oxygen — reactive species

CILIARY DYSKINESIS

Alternative but more adequate name for the immotile cilia syndrome. Three major forms can be distinguished by electron microscopy: defective dynein arms, defective radial spokes and microtubule translocation (8 plus 2 defect). This categorization clarifies why some patients suffering from the syndrome have spermatozoa with some degree of motility.

1. Zamboni, L. (1992). Sperm structure and its relevance to infertility. An electron microscopic study. *Arch. Pathol. Lab. Med.*, 116(4), 325

Related subjects: immotile cilia syndrome, Kartagener's syndrome, morphology — abnormal and normal

CLOMIPHENE CITRATE

A synthetic non-steroidal anti-estrogen that is structurally related to diethylstilbestrol (DES). Its therapeutic role in male infertility is still controversial since evaluation of well designed studies shows only non-significant effects. Patients with elevated follicle stimulating hormone (FSH) levels, severe oligo-asthenoteratozoospermia or azoospermia and those with very abnormal testicular biopsy are unlikely to respond to clomiphene citrate therapy. The usual prescribed dose is 12.5–50 mg/day given continuously or on 25-day cycle with a 5-day rest period each month. Monitoring of serum testosterone level is essential during treatment as high levels have a negative effect on spermatogenesis.

1. Micic, S. and Dotlic, R. (1985). Evaluation of sperm parameters in clinical trial with clomiphene citrate of oligospermic men. *J. Urol.*, **133**, 221

2. O'Donovan, P., Vandekerchhove, P., Lilford, R. and Hughes, E. (1993). Treatment of male infertility. Is it effective? Review and meta analysis of published randomized controlled trials. *Hum. Reprod.*, **8**, 1209

3. World Health Organization (1992). A double-blind trial of clomiphene citrate for the treatment of idiopathic male infertility. *Int. J. Androl.*, **15**, 299

Related subjects: medication — treatment, tamoxifen

COMPUTER-ASSISTED SPERM ANALYSIS (CASA)

Computer-aided sperm analysis was introduced in 1985, CellSoft and CellTrak being the first systems to be available. Measurements are imprecise when the count is less than 20 million/ml or more than 50 million/ml sperm cells, or when debris or other than sperm cells are present. The consequence is that samples have to be concentrated, diluted or washed. CASA systems should be used for determination of the concentration of progressively motile spermatozoa and their movement characteristics (see Figure 9). The digitization threshold significantly affects CASA results, although there is no objective method to establish the optimal threshold. In addition, no general standards are followed within or between instruments. Until these

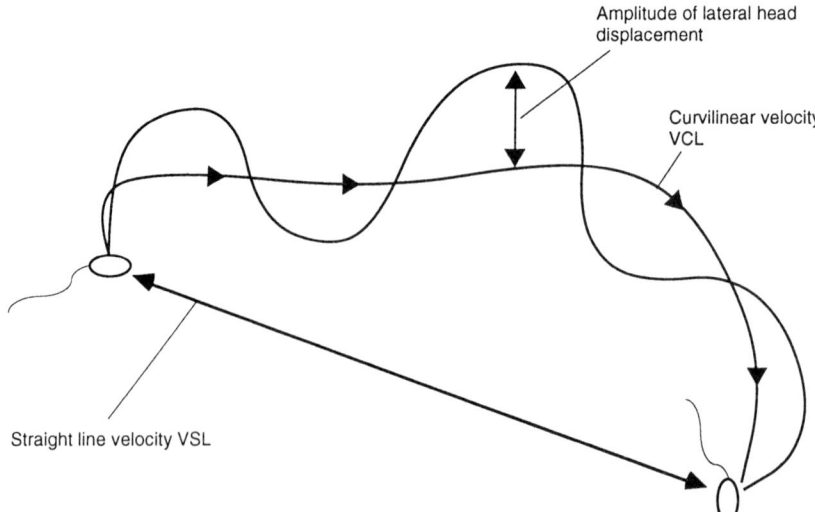

Amplitude of lateral head displacement

Curvilinear velocity VCL

Straight line velocity VSL

Figure 9 Computer-assisted analysis of sperm movement. The position of the head with respect to the body is followed and plotted. VCL = curvilinear velocity, VSL = straight-line velocity

problems are solved, CASA is often a research tool used for sperm motion parameters such as curvilinear velocity (VCL), straight-line velocity (VSL) and amplitude of lateral head displacement (ALH). Recently a morphology (head size) and a hyperactivation module have been introduced. For the time being these extensions suffer from the same problems as the other items, mainly a lack of standardization. Operator training and standardization of sample handling techniques can enhance reproducibility of CASA, although CASA measurements usually are more consistent than manual methods.

1. Davis, R.O. and Katz, D.F. (1992). Standardization and comparability of CASA instruments. *J. Androl.*, **13**, 81

2. Davis, R.O. and Katz, D.F. (1993). Operational standards for CASA instruments. *J. Androl.*, **14**, 385

3. Holt, W., Watson, P., Curry, M. and Holt, C. (1994). Reproducibility of computer-aided semen analysis: comparison of five different systems used in a practical workshop. *Fertil. Steril.*, **62**(6), 1277

4. Liu, D.Y., Clarke, A.N. and Gordon Baker, H.W. (1991). Relationship between sperm motility assesed with the Hamilton-Thorn motility analyzer and fertilization rates *in vitro. J. Androl.*, **12**, 231

5. Mortimer, D. (1990). Objective analysis of sperm motility and kinematics. In Keel. B.A. and Webster, B.W. (eds.) *Handbook of the Laboratory Diagnosis and Treatment of Infertility.* (Boca Raton: CRC Press)

Related subjects: semen analysis — normal values and predictive value

CONGENITAL ABSENCE OF VAS DEFERENS

The most common manifestation of the cystic fibrosis gene is congenital absence of the vas deferens. Findings may include bilateral or unilateral agenesis, complete or partial absence of the vas or of the cauda or the corpus of the epididymis. Depending on the genotype of the patient, pancreatic and/or lung symptoms are also present or may later develop. Genetic screening and counselling of affected males and their partners is therefore mandatory.

1. Lemna, W.K., Feldman, G.L. and Kerem, B. (1990). Mutation analysis for heterozygote detection and the prenatal diagnosis of cystic fibrosis. *N. Engl. J. Med.*, **322**, 291

2. Oates, R.D. and Amos, J.A. (1993). Congenital bilateral absence of the vas deferens and cystic fibrosis: a genetic commonality. *World J. Urol.*, **11**, 82

3. Oates, R.D. and Amos, J.A. (1994). The genetic basis of congenital bilateral absence of the vas deferens and cystic fibrosis. *J. Androl.*, **15**, 1

4. Wagenknecht, L.V. (1995). Alloplastic spermatocele. In Goldstein, M. (ed.) *Surgery for Male Infertility.* (Philadelphia: W.B. Saunders)

Related subjects: azoospermia, cystic fibrosis, microepididymal sperm aspiration, physical examination — male infertility, seminal vesicle, spermatocele — artificial, ultrasonography

CONGENITAL ADRENAL HYPERPLASIA (CAH)

A condition characterized by an inherited defect in the enzymes necessary for synthesis of cortisol with secondary excessive secretion of adrenocorticotropic hormone (ACTH) which results in adrenal hyperplasia and adrenal androgen overproduction. The most common enzymatic defect is 21-hydroxylase deficiency. Another, less common form is 3β-hydroxysteroid dehydrogenase deficiency. Male infertility may occur due to suppression of gonadotropins by excessive adrenal androgens which prevents testicular maturation and causes spermatogenesis failure. CAH has been associated with testicular tumors. The diagnosis of CAH can occur late (late onset CAH) and such patients may present initially with secondary infertility.

1. Augarten, A., Weissenberg, R., Pariente, C. and Sack, J. (1991). Reversible male infertility in late onset congenital adrenal hyperplasia. *J. Endocrinol. Invest.*, 14, 23

2. Keely, E.J., Matwijiw, I., Thliveris, J.A. and Faiman, C. (1993). Congenital adrenal hyperplasia with testicular tumors, aggression and gonadal failure. *Urology*, 41, 346

3. Srikant, M.S., West, B.R., Ishitani, M., Isaacs, H. Jr, Applebaum, H. and Costin, G. (1992). Benign testicular tumors in children with congenital adrenal hyperplasia. *J. Pediatr. Surg.*, 27, 639

Related subjects: genetics, hypogonadotropic hypogonadism

CREATINE KINASE

An enzyme which is important for sperm energy transport in spermatozoa. Increased amounts of creatine kinase (CK) have been associated with diminished fertilizing potential and with sperm cell immaturity. In sperm samples with high CK activity, abnormal morphology due to a higher retention of cytoplasm (cytoplasmatic droplets) has been reported.

1. Huszar, G., Vigue, L. and Corrales, M. (1990). Sperm creatine kinase activity in fertile and infertile oligospermic men. *J. Androl.*, 11(1), 40

2. Huszar, G. and Vigue, L. (1993). Incomplete development of human spermatozoa is associated with increased creatin phosphokinase concentration and abnormal head morphology. *Mol. Reprod. Dev.*, 34(30), 292

Related subjects: semen analysis — biochemical test of spermatozoa

CRYOPRESERVATION

Human spermatozoa have successfully been frozen since 1953. Generally there are two main categories of sperm freezing: for homologous and for heterologous (donor) use. Indications for homologous freezing are:

(1) Preservation of reproductive potential before chemotherapy, radiation therapy or surgery.

(2) Availability of spermatozoa at the time they are required for infertility treatment (*in vitro* fertilization, intrauterine insemination): absence of

husband, performance anxiety and previous poor specimen at on-demand occasions.

(3) Storage before vasectomy.

(4) Supernumerary spermatozoa after a surgical intervention to obtain spermatozoa (e.g. microsurgical epididymal sperm aspiration with *in vitro* fertilization and intracytoplasmic sperm injection).

Prediction of sperm recovery after freezing and thawing, the number of recovered motile spermatozoa, is possible by the application of computer-aided semen analysis to the prefreeze specimen. Straight-line velocity, linearity, curvilinear velocity and amplitude of lateral head displacement are the most common predictors. Successful cryopreservation is dependent on the rates of freezing, above and below the freezing point, and the composition of the solution in which the spermatozoa are frozen. To avoid damage due to cold-shock, protocols are used which freeze at slow rate from room temperature to the freezing point (1–2° per minute). For further protection, cryoprotectants and extenders are added to the freezing medium. Glycerol is the most successful cryoprotectant for sperm cryopreservation. It depresses the freezing point and reduces the electrolyte concentration to which sperm cells are exposed, maintains the pH and increases membrane stability. Extenders are additional compounds which assist the cryoprotectant by optimizing osmotic pressure and pH, and provide energy, thus avoiding intracellular phospholipid usage. Examples of extenders are dipolar buffers (TRIS, TES) and egg-yolk. Thawing is usually performed in a slow-thaw protocol in 20–35° air. If cryopreserved semen is employed for donor use, a strict protocol including screening for transmissible disease of each delivered specimen and a quarantine period to monitor possible seroconversion of the donor is mandatory. Screening ideally consists of serum testing for HIV, HBsAg, HBC and VDRL, semen culture including culture for gonorrhea and *Ureaplasma* and urethral *Chlamydia* testing.

1. American Fertility Society (1990). New guidelines for the use of donor semen insemination. *Fertil. Steril.*, 53(3), Suppl.

2. Bunge, R.G. and Sherman, J.K. (1953). Fertilizing capacity of frozen human spermatozoa. *Nature*, 172, 767

3. Davis, R.O., Drobnis, E.Z. and Overstreet, J.W. (1995). Application of multivariate cluster, discriminate function, and stepwise regression ananlysis to variable selection and predictive modeling of sperm cryosurvival. *Fertil. Steril.*, 63(5), 1051

4. Mahadevan, M. and Trounson, A.O. (1984). Effect of cooling, freezing and thawing rates and storage conditions on preservation of human spermatozoa. *Andrologia*, 16, 52

5. Sherman, J.K. (1990). Cryopreservation of human semen. In Keel, B.A. and Webster, B.W. (eds.) *Handbook of the Laboratory Diagnosis and Treatment of Infertility*. (Boca Raton: CRC Press)

Related subjects: computer-aided semen analysis, insemination

CRYPTORCHIDISM

Literally, this means that there is an impalpable testis, but usually it is referred to as an undescended testicle. It is a developmental defect characterized by some degree of failure of the testis to descend into the scrotum. The incidence in newborns is 3–5%, of which 15% is bilateral; at 9 months the rate is less than 1%. If bilateral, it is associated with severely reduced fertility secondary to oligoasthenozoospermia. The prognosis is somewhat better if the maldescent is unilateral. Of the men that underwent unilateral orchidopexy at an average age of 7–9 years, 80% fathered a child compared to 30% of those with bilateral orchidopexy. One of the determinants for the prognosis in case of cryptorchidism seems to be the scrotal temperature: the mean temperature of an undescended testis is 34.4°C, the temperature of a normal descended testicle was 33.2°C. The effect of early treatment is still debatable. Although the best time of treatment has not yet been defined, there is evidence that the child should be older than 9 months (as up till this time spontaneous descent can occur), but younger than 2 years. Treatment may consist of hormonal therapy (luteinizing hormone releasing hormone agonists with or without human chorionic gonadotropin) alone or as a preoperative preparation for orchidopexy.

1. Anonymous (1994). Aetiology of testicular cancer: association with congenital abnormalities, age at puberty, infertility, and exercise. United Kingdom Testicular Cancer Study Group. *Br. Med. J.*, **308**, 1393

2. Cendron, M., Keating, M.A. and Huff, D.S. (1989). Cryptorchidism, orchiopexy and infertility: a critical longterm retrospective analysis. Part II. *J. Urol.*, **142**, 559

3. Lee, P. (1993). Fertility in cryptorchidism. Does treatment make a difference? *Endocrinol. Metab. Clin. N. Am.*, **22**(3), 479

4. Mieusset, R., Bujan, L., Massat, G., Mansat, A. and Pontonnier, F. (1995). Clinical and biological characteristics of infertile men with a history of cryptorchidism. *Hum. Reprod.*, **10**(3), 613

5. Rozanski, T.A. and Bloom, D.A. (1995). The undescended testis. Theory and management. In Kaplan G.W. (ed.) Common problems in pediatric urology. *Urol. Clin. N. Am.*, **22**(1), 107

Related subjects: antisperm antibodies, diethylstilboestrol, epispadia, history — male infertility, human chorionic gonadotropin, hypospadia, Kallmann's syndrome, Klinefelter's syndrome, Noonan's syndrome, orchidopexy, physical examination — male infertility, retractile testis, scrotal temperature, spermatogenic arest, testicular cancer

CULTURE MEDIA, FOR HUMAN SPERMATOZOA

The major component in culture media is water. Three types of water can be distinguished:

(1) Tap water, as supplied locally.

(2) Reagent water, double- or more distilled, deionized or purified by reverse osmosis. No attention is paid towards sterility.

(3) Highly purified tissue culture water, grade I and II. The use of this water is essential in reproductive laboratories.

A selection of more commonly used media is given in Table 8. An important issue is the question of how to protect gametes and embryos for damage due to reactive oxygen species during handling procedures in culture medium. Most likely circumstances will approach more physiological conditions when anti-oxidants are substituted to the media.

Table 8 The uses of the more commonly used culture media for human spermatozoa

Name	Use	Comment
Phosphate buffered saline (PBS)	IUI	basic sperm preparation medium- no nutrients; cannot support capacitation in lengthy culture
Earle's balanced salt solution (EBSS)	IUI/IVF	common in IVF labs
Biggers, Whittens, Whittingham (BWW)	IUI/IVF	not generally used now; was utilized in animal work
Human tubal fluid (HTF)	IUI/IVF	common in IVF labs
Tyrodes modified T6	IUI/IVF	largely replaced by EBSS or HTF
Menezo B2 and B3	IUI/IVF	commercial: opinions vary in literature regarding efficiency
Ham's F10	IUI/IVF	controversial due to iron content

IUI = intrauterine insemination, IVF = *in vitro* fertilization

1. Biggers, J.D., Whitten, W.K. and Whittingham, D.G. (1971). The culture of mouse embryos *in vitro*. In Daniel, J.C. (ed.) *Methods in Mammalian Embryology*. (San Francisco: WH Freeman)

2. Menezo, Y., Testart, J. and Perrone, D. (1984). Serum is not necessary in human *in vitro* fertilization in huamn *in vitro* fertilization, early embryo culture, and transfer. *Fertil. Steril.*, 42, 750

3. Nishimoto, T., Yamada, I., Niwa, K., Mori, T., Nishimura, T. and Iritani, A. (1982). Sperm penetration *in vitro* human oocytes matured in a chemically defined medium. *J. Reprod. Fertil.*, 64, 115

4. Purdy, J.M. (1982). Methods for fertilization and embryo culture *in vitro*. In Edwards, R.G. and Purdy, J.M. (eds.) *Human Conception In Vitro*. (London: Academic Press)

5. Quinn, P.J., Kerin, J.F. and Warnes, G.M. (1985). Improved pregnancy rate in human *in vitro* fertilization with the use of a medium based on the composition of human tubal fluid. *Fertil. Steril.*, 44, 493

6. Quinn, P.J., Warnes, G.M., Kerin, J.F. and Kirby, C. (1984). Culture factors in relation to the success of human *in vitro* fertilization and embryo transfer. *Fertil. Steril.*, 41, 202

7. Tarin, J., de los Santos, M.J., de Oliveira, M.N.M., Pellicer, A. and Bonilla-Musole, F. (1994). Ascorbate supplemented media in short term cultures of human embryo's. *Hum. Reprod.*, 9, 1717

Related subjects: anti-oxidants, oxygen — reactive species, sperm preparation, taurine

CULTURE, SEMEN

Although infections of the male genital tract and the seminal fluid often show leukocytospermia, the presence of leukocytes is not specific for infection. Therefore, if leukocytes are present, a microbiological culture should be routine. In this context it should be noted that a high pH and the presence of lysozymes and zinc are bactericidal. In addition, not all cultured organisms are pathological or related to infertility. Micro-organisms considered to be part of the normal flora of the male reproductive tract include, amongst others, enterococci such as *Streptococcus faecalis* and staphylococci like *Staphylococcus epidermidis*. Special precautions should, therefore, be taken to avoid contamination (e.g. voiding before the production of the semen sample, washing of hands and penis with soap and the use of a sterile container). Uniform growth of organisms such as *Escherichia coli*, *Streptococcus faecalis* or *Klebsiella* indicate infection. Culture of anaerobic bacteria is not useful, since they are rarely found and probably play no role in male infertility.

1. Comhaire, F.H., Vermeulen, L., Verschraegen, G. and Claeys, G. (1992). Bacteriology and leukospermia: diagnosis of male accessory gland infection. In Acosta, A.A. (ed.) *Human Spermatozoa in Assisted Reproduction.* (Baltimore: Williams and Wilkins)

2. World Health Organization (1992). *WHO Laboratory Manual for the Examination of Human Semen and Sperm–Cervical Mucus Interaction,* 3rd edn. (Cambridge: Cambridge University Press)

Related subjects: bacterial infection, leucocytospermia, prostatitis, semen analysis — collection of sample

CYSTIC FIBROSIS

Cystic fibrosis is an autosomal recessive disorder caused by abnormalities in the cystic fibrosis transmembrane conductance regulator gene (CFTR). CFTR encodes for a chloride channel that regulates secretion in many exocrine tissues. The clinical presentation of cystic fibrosis is therefore diverse. More than 400 mutations in the CFTR gene have been described. The type and nature of the mutation determines the phenotypical expression of this gene in the patient. Cystic fibrosis and congenital absence of the vas deferens (CAVD) represent both ends of the spectrum. CAVD is present in nearly all males with cystic fibrosis, whereas the presence of pancreatic and lung involvement depends on the type of mutation and/or environmental factors. In the case of CAVD, genetic screening of the couple is indicated.

1. Dean, M. and Santis, G. (1994). Heterogeneity in the severity of cystic fibrosis and the role of CFTR genes mutations. *Hum. Genet.*, **93**(4), 364

2. Lemna, W.K., Feldman, G.L. and Kerem, B. (1990). Mutation analysis for heterozygote detection and the prenatal diagnosis of cystic fibrosis. *N. Engl. J. Med.*, **322**, 291

3. Oates, R.D. and Amos, J.A. (1993). Congenital bilateral absence of the vas deferens and cystic fibrosis: a genetic commonality. *World J. Urol.*, **11**, 82

4. Oates, R.D. and Amos, J.A. (1994). The genetic basis of congenital bilateral absence of the vas deferens and cystic fibrosis. *J. Androl.*, **15**, 1

Related subjects: azoospermia, congenital absence of vas deferens, microepididymal sperm aspiration, Young's syndrome

D*d*

DIABETES MELLITUS

The literature is conflicting as to whether diabetic men have disturbances in their gonadotropin regulation or not. Variable levels are reported for luteinizing hormone, follicle stimulating hormone and testosterone. Semen parameters may also be suboptimal. Most manifestations of diabetes mellitus, except for sexual dysfunction, are related to the control of and the duration of the disease. Sexual dysfunction can be present in all its possible forms: reduced erection, impotence and libido disorders. In patients with organic sexual dysfunction, signs of gonadal dysfunction are often reflected in low free testosterone and high luteinizing hormone levels.

1. Dinulovic, D. and Radonjic, G. (1990). Diabetes mellitus and male infertility. *Arch. Androl.*, **25**(3), 277

2. Garcia-Diez, L.C., Corrales Hernandez, J.J., Hernandez-Diaz, J. and Miralles, J.M. (1991). Semen characteristics and diabetes mellitus. *Arch. Androl.*, **26**(2), 119

3. Murray, F.T., Wyss, H.U., Thomas, R.G., Spevack, M. and Glaros, A.G. (1987). Gonadal dysfunction in diabetic men with organic impotence. *J. Clin. Endocrinol. Metab.*, **65**, 127

Related subjects: candidiasis, hypergonadotropic hypogonadism, impotence, retrograde ejaculation, sexual dysfunction

DIETHYLSTILBESTROL (DES)

Exposure of the male fetus to maternal DES treatment in early pregnancy has been associated with an increased incidence of cryptorchidism, testicular hypoplasia and epididymal cysts. Affected males may have abnormal semen analysis and reduced fertility. Sperm density, count, motility and morphology are affected. The data for an increased risk for the development of testicular cancer are not conclusive.

1. Bibbo, M. and Gill, W.B. (1981). Screening of male adolescents exposed to diethylstilbestrol *in utero*. *Pediatr. Clin. N. Am.*, **28**, 379

2. Marselos, M. and Tomatis, L. (1992). Diethylstilbestrol: pharmacology, toxicology and carcinogenicity in humans. *Eur. J. Cancer*, **28A**(6-7), 1182

3. Stillman, R. (1982). *In utero* exposure to diethylstilbestrol: adverse effect on the reproductive tract and reproductive performance in male and female offspring. *Am. J. Obstet. Gynecol.*, **142**, 905

4. Whitehead, E.D. and Leither, E. (1981). Genital abnormalities and abnormal semen analysis in male patients exposed to diethylstilbestrol *in utero. J. Urol.*, 125, 47–50

Related subjects: cryptorchidism, history — male infertility, testicular cancer

DIRECT INTRAFOLLICULAR INSEMINATION (DIFI)

An assisted reproductive technique in which follicles after ovarian hyperstimulation are injected with a small volume of prepared semen under ultrasound guidance. The advantage of the method is that it is simple and does not require any cell culture system. As for its indications, it is comparable to direct intraperitoneal insemination, since it requires normal tubal function.

1. Lucena, E., Ruiz, J.A., Mendoza, J.C., Lucena, A., Lucena, C. and Arango, A. (1991). Direct intrafollicular insemination. A case report. *J. Reprod. Med.*, 36(7), 525

2. Nuojua-Huttunen, S., Tuomivaara, L., Juntunen, K., Tomas, C., Kaupila, A. and Martikainen, H. (1995). Intrafollicular insemination for the treatment of infertility. *Hum. Reprod.*, 10(1), 91

Related subjects: assisted reproduction

DIRECT INTRAPERITONEAL INSEMINATION (DIPI)

A procedure in which prepared spermatozoa are inseminated directly into the peritoneal cavity. It has been attempted in patients with infertility due to a cervical factor, unexplained infertility and male subfertility. Normal female tubal and ovarian function is a prerequisite. The indication in patients other than those with cervical factor is controversial. Its potential complications include risk of infection, ectopic pregnancy and, when superovulation is used, hyperstimulation and multiple pregnancy. Antisperm antibody formation is considered a theoretical risk, but it has not been proven clinically.

1. Campos-Liete, E., Insull, M., Kennedy, S.H., Ellis, J.D., Sargent, I. and Barlow, D.H. (1992). A controlled assessment of direct intraperitoneal insemination [see comments]. *Fertil. Steril.*, 57, 168

2. Crosignani, P.G., Ragni, G., Finzi, G.C., De Lauretis, L., Olivares, M.D. and Perotti, L. (1991). Intraperitoneal insemination in the treatment of male and unexplained infertility. *Fertil. Steril.*, 55, 333

3. Crosignani, P.G. (1993). Lack of immunization after intraperitoneal insemination of spermatozoa. *Andrologia*, 25, 3

Related subjects: assisted reproduction

DOWN'S SYNDROME

Usually males with trisomy 21, Down's syndrome, have a mild degree of testicular dysfunction. The levels of luteinizing hormone are usually elevated; those of follicle stimulating hormone may vary. Variable findings are present in testicular biopsy: reduction in germ cell content but Leydig cells are often normal (Sertoli cell-only syndrome).

1. Swersie, S., Hueckel, J., Hudson, B. and Paulsen, C.A. (1971). Endocrine, histologic and genetic features of the hypogonadism in patients with Down's syndrome. *53rd Annual Meeting of the Endocrine Society*, San Francisco, abstract 440

Related subjects: hypergonadotropic hypogonadism

DRUG ABUSE

The harmful effects of a certain drug on reproduction are dependent on the type of drug (Table 9), the amount taken, the frequency and the length of the abuse and the age of the user.

Table 9   The effects of different illegal drugs on the male reproductive system

Class + drug	Endocrine	Semen
CNS depressant: marijuana, tetra-hydrocannabinol	inhibit secretion of FSH, LH and PRL, low T?	decreased testicular size degenerative spermatogenesis abnormal morphology decreased motility
CNS stimulant/ local anesthetic: cocaine	low dose leads to LH increase, but high dose inhibits LH release	topical: prolonged erection and delayed ejaculation aphrodisiac
Narcotics: heroin morphine, methadone	controversial reports on FSH, LH and T	atrophy accessory sex organs decreased fertility

FSH = follicle stimulating hormone, LH = luteinizing hormone, PRL = prolactin, T = testosterone

1. Smith, C.G. and Asch, R.H. (1987). Drug abuse and reproduction. *Fertil. Steril.*, 48(33) 55

Related subjects: history — male infertility, medication — negative effects, sexual function — drugs interfering

E*e*

EJACULATE, COMPOSITION

Contributions to the ejaculate volume by the different male accessory glands are as follows:

(1) Cowper and Littre glands 3–5%;

(2) Epididymis 5–10%;

(3) Seminal vesicle 50–70%;

(4) Prostate 15–30%;

(5) Spermatozoa 1–5%.

Related subjects: anatomy, epididymis, prostate, seminal vesicle, sperm maturation, split ejaculate

EJACULATORY DUCT OBSTRUCTION

The ejaculatory duct consists of a tract 2 cm in length formed by the union of the ampulla of the vas deferens and the duct of the seminal vesicle, after which it enters the prostatic urethra. Obstruction should be suspected in patients with a possible history of infection, a low ejaculatory volume, azoospermia or a markedly reduced sperm count. A normal volume does not rule out obstruction. The obstruction may be complete or partial and be located high or low. The testicles are usually of normal size. Epididymal induration may be present. On transrectal ultrasonography, ejaculatory midline cysts or dilatation of the seminal vesicle or vasal ampulla may be seen. Transurethral incision or deroofing of a cyst of the ejaculatory ducts is the treatment of choice, although the improvement of semen quality after treatment is disappointing.

1. Gilbert, B.R. (1995). Transurethral resection for ejaculatory duct obstruction. In Goldstein, M. (ed.) *Surgery For Male Infertility*. (Philadelphia: W.B. Saunders)

2. Meacham, R.B., Hellerstein, D.K. and Lipshultz, L.I. (1993). Evaluation and treatment of ejaculatory duct obstruction in the infertile male. *Fertil. Steril.*, 59, 393

Related subjects: azoospermia, oligozoospermia/low volume — flowsheet, physical examination, ultrasonography, vasography

ELECTRO-EJACULATION

In patients with ejaculatory disorders, electro-ejaculation is an important therapeutical option. The probe is inserted into the rectum and pressure is applied in anterior direction. The voltage is slowly increased. Ninety percent of patients will produce an ejaculate with this method at less than 20 V and 50 stimulations. Modern rectal probes have built-in thermistors to avoid heat damage to the rectum. Some patients require anesthesia for the procedure. Preparation consists either of alkalinization of the urine with oral Na bicarbonate or catheterization with subsequent instillation of culture medium in the bladder.

1. Bennett, C.J., Ayers, J.W.T., Randolph, J.F., Seager, S.W.J., McCabe, M. and Moinipanah, R. (1988). Sexual function and electroejaculation in men with spinal cord injury: review. *J. Urol.*, **139**, 453

2. Brindley, G.S. (1981). Electroejaculation: its technique, neurological implication and uses. *J. Neurol. Neurosurg. Psychiatry*, **44**, 9

3. Witt, M. and Grantmyre, J. (1993). Ejaculatory failure. *World J. Urol.*, **11**, 89

Related subjects: anejaculation, paraplegia, spinal cord injury, vibratory stimulation

EMBRYOLOGY, MALE (Table 10)

Related subjects: agonadism, androgen insensitivity syndrome, anorchia, azoospermia factor, endocrinology, gonadal dysgenesis, gonadodysgenesis, Mullerian inhibiting factor, testicular feminization, testis determining factor, Y chromosome

ENDOCRINOLOGY

The reference values for some of the male reproductive hormones listed in Table 11 are given in Table 12. Spermatogenesis requires the action of follicle stimulating hormone on the tubular compartment, and of luteinizing hormone on the interstitial compartment and subsequent stimulation of testosterone production by the Leydig cells (see Figure 10). However, intratesticular control mechanisms, both autocrine (acting upon the cell which secreted it) and paracrine (affecting another neighbourhood cell) are involved in the regulation of testicular function as well. Listed below are some of the factors thought to be involved in the local control system (Table 13).

1. Niederberger, C.S., Shubhada, S., Kim, S.J. and Lamb, D.J. (1993). Paracrine factors and the regulation of spermatogenesis. *World J. Urol.*, **11**(2), 120

2. Veldhuis, J. (1991). The hypothalamic–pituitary–testicular axis. In Yen, S.S.C. and Jaffe, R.B. (eds.) *Reproductive Endocrinology*, 3rd edn. (Philadelphia: W.B. Saunders)

3. Verhoeven, G. (1992). Local control systems within the testis. *Bailliere's Clin. Endocrinol. Metab.*, **6**(2), 435

Table 10   The embryology of the male reproductive system

Gestational age (weeks)	Normal	Abnormal
4–6	Migration of bipotential primordial germ cells into gonadal ridge	failure of germ cell migration causes gonadal agenesis (streaks)
6	Bipotential stage of gonads: *germ cells *mesenchyme (theca–Leydig) *epithelium (granulosa–Sertoli) *mesonephric duct system	
6–8	In the presence of Y chromosome testicular determining factor (TDF) testicular development, differentiation of medulla and regression of cortex occurs. This involves: (1) Sertoli cells form spermatogenic cord and seminiferous tubules; and (2) Leydig cell formation	absence of TDF causes gonadal dysgenesis translocation of TDF causes XX males
8–9	Anti-Mullerian hormone (Mullerian inhibiting factor) secreted by Sertoli cells causes regression of Mullerian ducts	retention of Mullerian system if there is no functional testis
8*–12	Synthesis of testosterone in Leydig cells and paracrine signalling through diffusion induce differentiation of nearby Wolffian duct into epididymis, vas deferens and seminal vesicles	regression of Wolffian system if there is no testosterone around
9–14	Testosterone secretion and local conversion to dihydrotestosterone induce masculinization of external genitalia leading to: genital tubercle (penis); labioscrotal folds (scrotum); and urogenital sinus folds (penile urethra)	female external genitalia (no Y ovary present, absence of gonad, abnormal androgen receptor, 5α-reductase def.)

*shortly after 8 weeks

Table 11   The hormones involved in the male reproductive system

Hormone	Type	Origin	Action
GnRH (LHRH)	decapeptide	median eminence of hypothalamus; pulsatile secretion	stimulation of synthesis and secretion of α- and β-subunits of FSH and LH
FSH	glycoprotein of two subunits: α-subunit and FSH β-subunit	anterior pituitary pars distalis; pulsatile secretion (60–90 min)	stimulation of Sertoli cells; initiation of spermatogenesis
LH	glycoprotein of two subunits: α-subunit and LH β-subunit	anterior pituitary, pars distalis; pulsatile secretion (60–90 min)	regulation of testosterone biosynthesis in Leydig cell; maintenance of spermatogenesis
Prolactin	polypeptide	anterior pituitary, pars lateralis	potentiation of LH effect on Leydig cells
Testosterone	steroid	Leydig cells	maintenance of spermatogenesis; prehormone for estradiol and dihydrotestosterone
Estradiol	steroid	extraglandular (fat, liver, muscle) aromatization from testosterone and androstenedione; 20–25% secretion by Leydig cells	regulation of LH secretion and control of bioactivity for LH
Inhibin	glycoprotein; hetero-dimers in two forms: α-subunit + βA-(inhibin A) or βB-(inhibin B) subunit	Sertoli cells	inhibitor of FSH secretion by pituitary
Activin	glycoprotein; hetero-dimer is βA + βB (activin AB), two homodimers are βA + βA (activin A) and βB + βB (activin B)	Leydig cells	stimulation of FSH secretion (*in vitro?*)

Table 12   Reference values for hormones involved in the male reproductive system

Hormone	Plasma levels	Conversion factor to SI units
FSH	1–7 mIU/ml	1 (IU/l)
LH	1–8 mIU/ml	1 (IU/l)
Testosterone	300–1200 ng/dl	10–40 nmol/l (0.0347)
Prolactin	1–20 ng/ml	45–800 pmol/l (44.4)
Estradiol		0–250 pmol/l (3.67)

FSH = follicle stimulating hormone, LH = luteinizing hormone

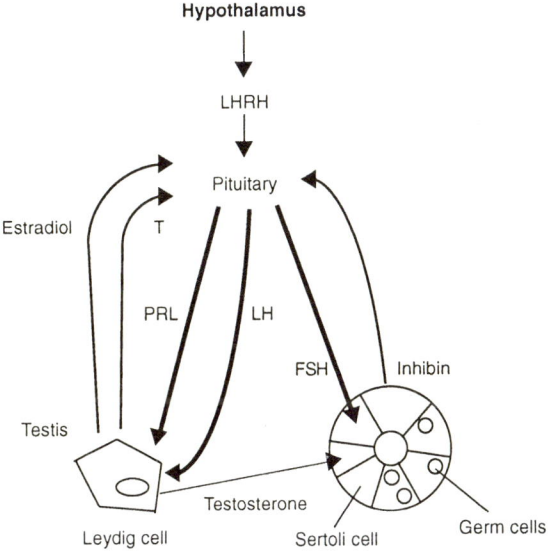

Figure 10   The interaction of different hormones involved in male reproduction. LHRH = luteinizing hormone releasing hormone, T = testosterone, PRL = prolactin, LH = luteinizing hormone, FSH = follicle stimulating hormone

Table 13   Testicular factors controlling spermatogenesis

Group	Substance
Peptide hormones	angiotensin II, atrial natriuretic peptide, oxytocin, vasopressin
Steroids	androgens, estrogens
Growth factors	activin, inhibin, insulin-like growth factor 1 (IGF-1), transforming growth factor (TGF) α and β
Releasing hormones	gonadotropin releasing hormone, corticotropin releasing factor
Cytokines	interleukin-1, interleukin-2

Related subjects: activin, androgen binding protein, estradiol, follicle stimulating hormone, gonadotropin releasing hormone, human chorionic gonadotropin, inhibin, luteinizing hormone, prolactin, testosterone, testosterone–estradiol binding globulin

EPIDIDYMIS

The epididymis consists of one long stretched tubule located on the dorsolateral side of the testicle and can be functionally divided into three main parts:

The caput (head)

A main function is concentration of viable spermatozoa up to 100-fold by resorption of testicular fluid and of spermatozoa of lesser quality.

The corpus (body)

Post-testicular maturation is an important feature of this section. Progressive motility is acquired, cytoplasmic droplets are lost, the final steps in the development of the acrosomal reaction occur and fertilizing ability is advanced.

The cauda (tail)

The proximal part is formed by ductuli efferentes, the distal one by the epididymal ducts. A main feature is sperm storage, since some 70% of the spermatozoa are stored here. In addition, spermatozoa of poor quality are resorbed. It is estimated that one-half of the spermatozoa released from the testis are resorbed by the epidymal epithelium. With prolonged storage, fertilizing capacity is lost initially, followed by motility and finally viability. Caudal spermatozoa are also sensitive to elevated scrotal temperature.

1. Mortimer, D. (1994). *Practical Laboratory Andrology*. (Oxford: Oxford University Press)

Related subjects: anatomy, ejaculate — composition, sperm maturation, semen analysis — biochemical test of seminal plasma

EPISPADIA

The opening of the urethra is located on the dorsal side of the penis. Often this congenital abnormality is associated with exstrophy of the bladder. Etiological factors in male infertility in these patients include cryptorchidism, erectile dysfunction, retrograde ejaculation, recurrent epididymo-orchitis and dysfunctional urethral transport. A low spontaneous pregnancy rate of around 20% is reported. Therapy may include reconstructive surgery and assisted reproductive techniques, depending on the availability and the quality of sperm. The incidence of the condition in combination with bladder exstrophy is 1 in 30 000 live births; as an isolated event this is 1 in 90 000 births.

1. Bastuba, M.D., Alper, M.M. and Oates, R.D. (1993). Fertility and the use of assisted reproductive techniques in the adult male exstrophy/epispadia patient. *Fertil. Steril.*, 60(4), 733

2. Hashmat, A.I. and Das, S. (1993). *The Penis*. (Philadelphia: Lea and Febiger)

Related subjects: cryptorchidism, retrograde ejaculation

ESTRADIOL

This is an estrogenic steroid hormone that in the male, together with estrone, is mainly obtained through extraglandular aromatization from testosterone and androstenedione. This conversion takes place in fat tissue, in the liver and in muscles. Secretion by Leydig cells accounts for around 20% of the estrogen production in men, the adrenal contributes less than 5%.

1. Veldhuis, J. (1991). The hypothalamic–pituitary–testicular axis. In Yen, S.S.C. and Jaffe, R.B. (eds.) *Reproductive Endocrinology*. (Philadelphia: W.B. Saunders)

Related subjects: endocrinology, Leydig cell

F*f*

FERTILIZATION

This is the process commonly referred to as the penetration of a mature oocyte by a functional spermatozoon, resulting in the formation of pronuclei (see Figure 11). However, fertilization cannot be said to be complete until syngamy occurs (i.e. fusion and exchange of genetic material between male and female gametes). This finally results in the formation of the zygote. The human sperm midpiece provides the centrosome necessary for further development to zygote and early embryo. Furthermore, successful fertilization does not indicate the ability of a zygote to undergo subsequent cleavage and blastulation. It should be realized that polyspermy and polygyny are also (abnormal) forms of fertilization. Capacitation and acrosome reaction are *in vivo* prerequisites for the ability of spermatozoa to penetrate the zona pellucida, leading to activation of the oocyte at the moment of contact between the sperm head and the oolemma.

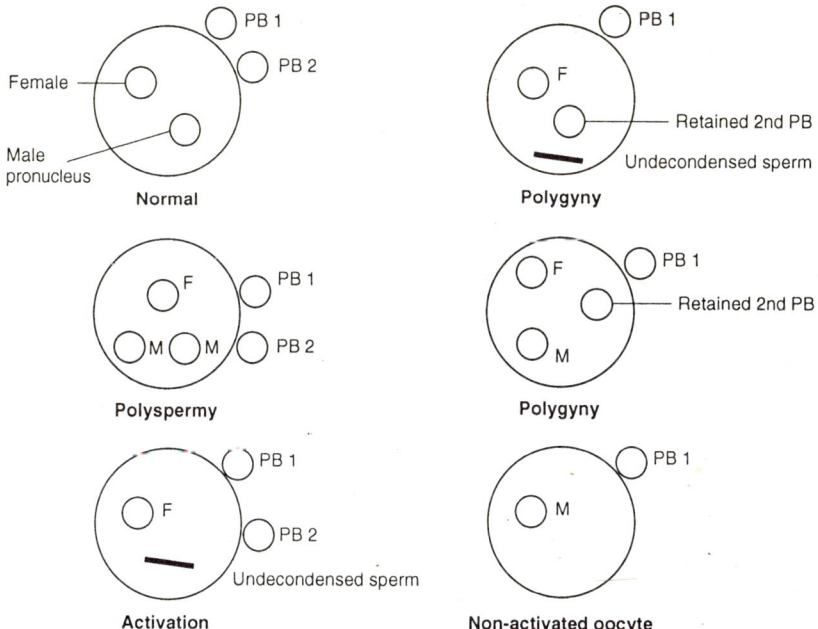

Figure 11   Normal and abnormal forms of fertilization. PB = polar body

1. Acosta, A.A. (1994). Process of fertilization in the human and its abnormalities: diagnostic and therapeutic possibilities. *Obstet. Gynecol. Surv.*, 49(8), 567–76

2. Bedford, J.M. (1994). The contraceptive potential of fertilization: a physiological perspective. *Hum. Reprod.*, 9(2), 52

Related subjects: acrosome reaction, capacitation

FLOW CYTOMETRY

Measures and categorizes individual cells in cell suspensions (e.g. spermatozoa). Cells pass in single file through a narrow laser beam. Subpopulations can be plotted as histograms according to viability, size, shape, DNA content (i.e. X–Y bearing), cell surface marking (acrosomal state, antibodies) and RNA content allowing for more objective and reproducable analysis. A fluorescent stain has to be applied such as fluorescein (stains protein) or acridine orange (stains DNA and RNA).

1. Spano, M. and Evenson, D.P. (1993). Flow cytometric analysis for reproductive biology. *Biol. Cell.*, 78(1-2), 53

Related subjects: acrosome reaction — test, lectins, semen analysis — biochemical tests of spermatozoa, sex selection, stains

FOLLICLE STIMULATING HORMONE (FSH)

FSH is a glycoprotein consisting of two subunits: one α-subunit and one FSH β-subunit. It is produced and secreted in the pars distalis of the anterior pituitary. Secretion is pulsatile, coupled to that of luteinizing hormone, with a pulse frequency of 60–90 minutes. The main function is stimulation of Sertoli cells, which in turn stimulate several proteins, androgen binding protein being one of the major ones. FSH is necessary for the initiation of spermatogenesis, and therefore if spermatogenesis has to be established, e.g. in a hypogonadotropic situation, treatment has to consist of both FSH (human menopausal gonadotropin) and luteinizing hormone (human chorionic gonadotropin) until spermatogenesis is established.

1. Veldhuis, J. (1991). The hypothalamic–pituitary–testicular axis. In Yen, S.S.C. and Jaffe, R.B. (eds.) *Reproductive Endocrinology*, 3rd edn. (Philadelphia: W.B. Saunders)

Related subjects: endocrinology, medication — treatment, Sertoli cell

FOLLICULAR FLUID

A protein rich mixture of plasma exudates and granulosa cell secretions providing nourishment and a specific endocrine micro-environment for the maturing oocyte. It promotes hyperactivation of the spermatozoa and aids in capacitation. It is controversial whether or not it can induce acrosomal reaction.

1. Hong, C.Y., Chao, H.T., Lee, S.L. and Wei, Y.H. (1993). Modification of human sperm function by follicular fluid: a review. *Int. J. Androl.*, 16(2), 93

Related subjects: acrosome reaction, capacitation, hyperactivation

Gg

GAMETE INTRAFALLOPIAN TRANSFER (GIFT)

A technique of assisted reproduction in which oocytes are aspirated from stimulated ovaries, mixed with capacitated sperm and replaced into one or two healthy Fallopian tubes, either by lapararoscopy or by ultrasound guided transcervical approach. The procedure is used as an alternative to *in vitro* fertilization and replacement of embryos in the uterine cavity, hence there is no need for advanced laboratory facilities. The procedure is less suitable for male infertility unless fertilizing potential has been demonstrated. Results of prospective randomized studies generally fail to show a favorable result for intratubal procedures, including comparison with intrauterine transfers.

1. Amso, N.N. and Shaw, R.W. (1993). A critical appraisal of assisted reproduction techniques. *Hum. Reprod.*, 8, 168

2. Asch, R.H. (1989). GIFT: indications, results, problems and perspectives. In Capitanio, G.L., Asch, R.H., De Cecco, L. and Croce, S. (eds.) *GIFT: Basis to Clinics*. (New York: Raven Press)

3. Asch, R.H., Ellsworth, L.R., Balmaceda, J.P. and Wong, P.C. (1984). Pregnancy after translaparoscopic gamete intrafallopian transfer (GIFT). *Lancet*, ii, 1034

Related subjects: assisted reproduction

GENDER

The gender identity is the sex with which an individual identifies himself or herself. It includes all behavior with any sexual connotation and is the end result of, primarily, genetic sex, and secondarily, the gonadal sex differentiation, including internal and external genitalia. In addition, the secondary sex characteristics appearing at puberty under the influence of hormone production and the role assigned by society in response to all above manifestations of sex contribute to the individual's identification.

GERM CELL MUTAGENS

The capacity of environmental agents, ionizing radiation and some mutagenic chemicals to induce transmissable genetic damage in germ cells has been clearly demonstrated in animals. Increased frequencies of chromosomal aberrations are detected in human spermatozoa following exposure to ionizing radiation or chemotherapeutic agents, but transmission of such induced alterations has not been demonstrated.

1. Doll, R., Evans, H.J. and Darby, S.C. (1994). Paternal exposure not to blame. *Nature*, **367**, 678

2. Shelby, M.D., Bishop, J.B., Mason, J.M. and Tindall, K.R. (1993). Fertility, reproduction and genetic disease: studies on the mutagenic effects of environmental agents on mammalian germ cells. *Environ. Health Perspect.*, **100**, 283

3. Shelby, M.D. (1994). Human germ cell mutagens. *Environ. Mol. Mutagen.*, **23** (Suppl. 24), 30

Related subjects: chemotherapy, chromosomal abnormalities — sperm cells, pesticides, radiation

GLOBOZOOSPERMIA

A form of abnormal sperm morphology in which the acrosome is completely absent. This gives the spermatozoon a round shape (see Figure 12); thus the defect is also called round head syndrome. Apart from the acrosomal agenesis, these sperm cells also have abnormal immature chromatin. The abnormality develops as a consequence of an abnormal topographical relationship between the Golgi apparatus and the spermatid nucleus. It is a congenital abnormality with a polygenic inheritance. Affected men are sterile when all of the spermatozoa show the abnormality. Recently, the first pregnancy was reported after employing intracytoplasmic sperm injection.

1. Trokoudes, K.M., Danos, N., Kaligirou, L., Vlachou, R., Lysiotis, T., Georghiadis, N. and Lerios, L. (1995). Pregnancy with spermatozoa from a globozoospermic man after intracytoplasmatic sperm injection treatment. *Hum. Reprod.*, **10**(4), 880

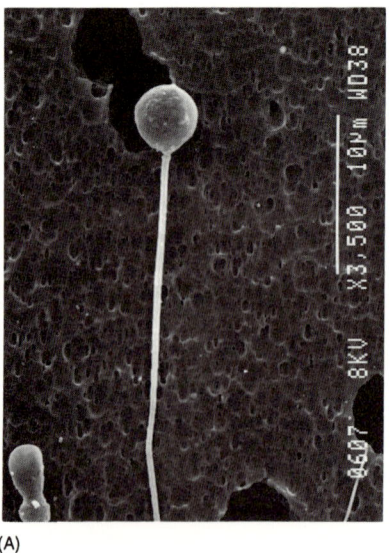 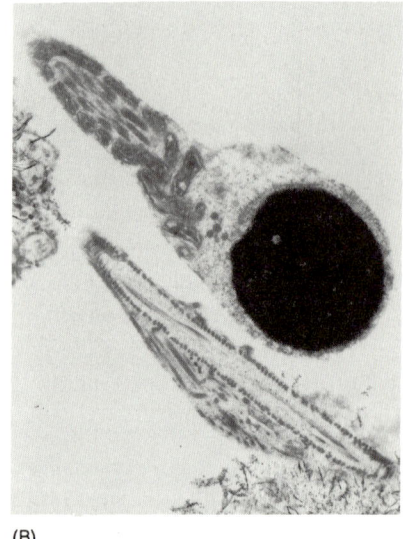

(A)   (B)

Figure 12 Globozoospermia shown on a scanning electron micrograph (SEM) (A) and transmission electron micrograph (B). The sperm shown in the SEM lack a midpiece

2. Zamboni, L. (1992). Sperm structure and its relevance to infertility. An electron microscopic study. *Arch. Pathol. Lab. Med.*, 116(4), 325

Related subjects: acrosome reaction, morphology abnormal and normal, teratozoospermia

GONADAL DYSGENESIS, PURE

These patients often present without Turner stigmata. They have female external genitalia, a uterus with Fallopian tubes, 46 XY karyotype, streak gonads, elevated gonadotropins, female androgen levels and low estrogens. The etiology is very early fetal testicular regression before 43 days after conception, probably due to a short arm deletion of the testis determining factor (TDF) gene or other chromosomal aberrations.

1. Berkovitz, G.D., Fechner, P.Y., Zacur, H.W., Rock, J.A., Snyder, H.M., Migeon, C.J. and Perlman, E.J. (1991). Clinical and pathological spectrum of 46 XY gonadal dysgenesis: its relevance to the understanding of sex differentiation. *Medicine*, 70, 375

2. Speroff, L., Glass, R.H. and Kase, N.G. (1993). *Clinical Gynecologic Endocrinology and Infertility*, 5th edn. (Baltimore: Williams and Wilkins)

Related subjects: agonadism, anorchia, embryology, gonadodysgenesis, hypergonadotropic hypogonadism

GONADODYSGENESIS (Table 14)

Normal development of testis and subsequently normal male outgrowth requires normal 46 XY chromosomal constitution and the presence of spermatogonia. Errors leading to testicular regression can occur at different times during pregnancy, because of chromosomal aberrations or as a result

Table 14   The different types of testicular gonadodysgenesis

Time of testicular regression in postconception days	Name	Mullerian ducts	Wolffian ducts	External genitalia
Before 43	pure gonadal dysgenesis	+	–	female
43–59	Swyer syndrome	+	–	female
60–69	agonadism	+	–	ambiguous
70–75	testicular dysgenesis	+	+	ambiguous
75–84	testicular regression	–	+	ambiguous
90–120	rudimentary testis	–	+	male
>140	anorchia – vanishing testis	–	+	male

of incidental calamity. All these syndromes have the following in common: a chromosomal constitution of 46 XY, the gonadal designation is testicular and, ultimately, the condition is characterized by elevated follicle stimulating hormone and luteinizing hormone.

1. Speroff, L., Glass, R.H. and Kase, N.G. (1993). *Clinical Gynecologic Endocrinology and Infertility*, 5th edn. (Baltimore: Williams and Wilkins)

Related subjects: agonadism, anorchia, embryology, gonadal dysgenesis, hypergonadotropic hypogonadism

GONADOTROPIN RELEASING HORMONE (GnRH)

GnRH, previously called luteinizing hormone releasing hormone (LHRH), is a decapeptide produced in the arcuate nucleus of the medial basal hypothalamus. It is secreted in a pulsatile manner at a frequency of 60–100 minutes. It stimulates the synthesis and the secretion of α- and β-subunits of follicle stimulating hormone and luteinizing hormone.

In male hypothalamic hypogonadotropic hypogonadism, theoretically the most physiological means of stimulating gonadotropic activity is pulsatile administration of GnRH. This can be performed either subcutaneously or intravenously through portable infusion pumps. The usual dose varies from 5 to 30 μg per 2 hours. There is controversy as to whether this approach yields better results than administration of gonadotropins. Direct comparison of pulsatile GnRH and human chorionic gonadotropin (hCG)/human menopausal gonadotropin (hMG) therapy in randomized trials has not revealed any advantages of GnRH. It is possible that a so-far unidentified subgroups of patients with normal gonadotropin levels but hormonal dysregulation may benefit from GnRH therapy.

1. Aulitzky, W., Frick, J. and Hadziselimovic, F. (1989). Pulsatile LHRH therapy in patients with oligozoospermia and disturbed luteinizing hormone pulsatility. *Int. J. Androl.*, **12**, 265

2. Liu, L., Banks, S.M., Barnes, K.M. and Sherins, R.J. (1988). Two-year comparison of testicular responses to to pulsatile gonadotropin-releasing hormone and exogenous gonadotropins from the inception of therapy in men with isolated hypogonadotropic hypogonadism. *J. Clin. Endocrinol. Metab.*, **67**, 140

3. Santen, R.J. (1991). Male hypogonadism. In Yen, S.S.C. and Jaffe, R.B. (eds.) *Reproductive Endocrinology*, 3rd edn. (Philadelphia: W.B. Saunders)

4. Schopohl, J., Mehltretter, G. and Zumbusch, R.V. (1991). Comparison of gonadotropin-releasing hormone and gonadotropin therapy in male patients with idiopathic hypogonadotropic hypogonadism. *Fertil. Steril.*, **56**, 1143

Related subjects: endocrinology, hypogonadotropic hypogonadism, medication — treatment

GONOCOCCAL INFECTION

Sexually transmitted disease caused by *Neisseria gonorrhoeae*. In males there is usually symptomatic urethritis, although as much as 2–5% of patients may be asymptomatic. Occasionally epididymitis and prostatitis occurs, resulting in obstructive azoospermia. Twenty to thirty per cent of patients have concomittant *Chlamydia trachomatis* infection. Therefore, treatment for gonorrhea should include treatment for *Chlamydia*. Because of the widespread occurrence of resistance of *gonococci* to antibiotics, all infections have to be treated as such. Recommendations include third generation cephalosporins (ceftriaxone 125/250 mg i.m., cefotaxime 500/1000 mg i.m.), quinolones (ciprofloxacin 500 mg, norfloxacin 800 mg), oral cephalosporins (cefixime 400 mg, cefuroxime axetil 1 g plus probenecid 1 g) or spectinomycin 2 g i.m.

1. Zenilman, J.M. (1992). Update on bacterial sexually transmitted disease. In Mellinger, B.C. and Smith, A.D. (eds.) *Urol. Clin. N. Am.*, 19(1), 25

Related subjects: *Chlamydia*, sexually transmitted diseases

GROWTH HORMONE (GH)

Growth hormone has a direct effect on Leydig cell function. In addition, pubertal maturation of the testis is determined by GH as well as gonadotropins. Co-treatment with GH of men with hypogonadotropic hypogonadism and azoospermia produced an augmented response to gonadotropins, probably resulting from an increase in insulin-like growth factor (IGF-1) production by GH.

1. Shoham, Z., Zalel, Y. and Jacobs, H.S. (1994). The role of growth hormone in male infertility. *Clin. Endocrinol.*, 41, 1

Related subjects: hypogonadotropic hypogonadism

H*h*

HEMATOSPERMIA

This is red coloration of the seminal fluid because of the presence of blood. The following causes have to be excluded: malignancy (15%), infection (30%), and prostatic calculi (20%). In about 15% of cases, no abnormality can be found.

1. Papp, G.K., Hoznek, A., Hegedus, M. and Juhasz, E. (1994). Hematospermia. *J. Androl.*, 15, 31S

Related subjects: asthenozoospermia, semen analysis — physical properties

HEMIZONA BINDING TEST

Human oocytes are dissected into halves, each half being exposed to the spermatozoa from the person being tested and a fertile control. The numbers of spermatozoa from the patient and the controls that bound to the zona are calculated and the ratio given. The test has shown a good correlation with *in vitro* fertilization results. Although oocytes can be stored in highly concentrated salt solution without affecting sperm binding and penetration of the zona pellucida, the main problem of the test is the limited availability of human oocytes.

1. Oehninger, S., Franken, D., Alexander, N. and Hodgen, G.D. (1992). Hemizona assay and its impact on the identification and treatment of human sperm. *Andrologia*, 24(6), 307–21

Related subjects: sperm function tests

HENDRY SCHEDULE

In men with antisperm antibodies different corticoid regimens have been tried in order to reduce the titer of antisperm antibodies. The high-dose regimen, usually referred to as the Hendry schedule, was abandoned because of serious side effects.

1. Hendry, W.F. (1982). Bilateral aseptic necrosis of femoral heads following intermittent high dose steroid therapy. *Fertil. Steril.*, 38, 120

Related subjects: antisperm antibodies — treatment, corticosteroids

HISTORY, IN MALE INFERTILITY

Evaluation of male infertility begins with a complete history (Table 15).

Table 15 Factors to be considered when taking a complete history from a man who presents with possible infertility

Personal	age duration of infertility primary or secondary profession(s)	
Family	congenital abnormalities infertility recurrent abortion	
Medical	illness	childhood (mumps, cryptorchism, onset puberty); systemic (TB); infections including urinary tract and sexually transmitted disease; scrotal trauma;
	treatments	drugs; surgery; radiation
Sexual	habits dysfunction	frequency of intercourse libido; erection; ejaculation
Toxins	lifestyle	clothing (underwear); heat (hot bath/sauna); smoking; coffee; alcohol
	occupational	gas, vapor, heavy metals, welding, radiation, heat, pesticides amount, duration
	drugs	

Related subjects: physical examination — male infertility

HYDROCELE

A usually painless accumulation of serous fluid between the visceral and the parietal layers of the tunica vaginalis. It can be congenital or acquired; in the latter case it is often associated with epididymitis or orchitis, but a tumor has to be ruled out. The fluid collection is in itself harmless and can be distinguished from a varicocele by its translucency, although chronic hydroceles sometimes are thick-walled and hence not translucent. There is no resulting decrease in sperm function and fertility.

1. Politoff, L., Hadziselimovic, F., Herzog, B. and Jenni, P. (1990). Does hydrocele affect later fertility? *Fertil. Steril.*, 53(4), 700–3

Related subjects: varicocele

HYPERACTIVATION

Hyperactivation is defined as an increased flagellar beat amplitude accompanied by decreased progressiveness of sperm movements *in vitro*. A circular-like movement is often seen which is also referred to as starspin movements. Hyperactivation occurs in the later part of the capacitation process, probably through opening of calcium channels in the sperm tail. The function of hyperactivated motility is suggested to be a necessity for sperm penetration of the cumulus oophorus, corona radiata and possibly penetration of the zona pellucida as well.

1. Suarez, S.S. and Pollard, J.W. (1990). Capacitation, the acrosome reaction and motility in mammalian sperm. In Gagnon, C. (ed.) *Controls of Sperm Motility: Biological and Clinical Aspects.* (Boca Raton: CRC Press)

Related subjects: capacitation, follicular fluid, sperm function tests, sperm maturation

HYPERGONADOTROPIC HYPOGONADISM

A term used for irreversible inability of the gonad (e.g. the testis) to produce gametes (e.g. spermatozoa) and it is signified by elevated follicle stimulating hormone (FSH) levels. The degree of elevation of FSH can be used as an index of the severity of germ cell dysfunction. The clinical presentation varies, depending on the age when the defect in testosterone secretion started. Primary disorders result in incomplete sexual maturation; in adults impotence is an early symptom. Fertility prognosis depends on the underlying cause as to whether spermatogenesis can be (re)established. Table 16 shows the most common etiologies.

Table 16   The most common etiologies of hypergonadotropic hypogonadism in men

Type of disorder	Examples
Chromosomal	Klinefelter's syndrome; myotonic dystrophy; XYY syndrome; Noonan's syndrome; Down's syndrome; translocations or deletions in which the SRY region is involved
Anatomic	agonadism; anorchia
Toxins	fungicides; heavy metals; radiation
Enzymatic	17α-hydroxylase deficiency; 17-keto-reductase deficiency
Orchitis	mumps; autoimmune
Diabetes mellitus	
Androgen insensitivity	
Luteinizing hormone resistance	

1. Santen, R.J. (1991). Male hypogonadism. In Yen, S.S.C. and Jaffe, R.B. (eds.) *Reproductive Endocrinology*, 3rd edn. (Philadelphia: W.B. Saunders)

Related subjects: agonadism, anorchia, androgen insentivity, congenital adrenal hyperplasia, diabetes mellitus, Down's syndrome, Klinefelter's syndrome, Noonan's syndrome, mumps, occupational hazards, pesticides, radiation

HYPERPROLACTINEMIA

Patients with hyperprolactinemia have normal or low gonadotropins and low testosterone levels. The mechanism in which it causes hypogonadotropism can result from direct action of prolactin on the hypothalamus resulting in dysregulation of gonadotropin releasing hormone and hence luteinizing hormone release. Another possibility is indirect action through pressure in the hypothalamic or pituitary area. Hyperprolactinemia is associated with both decreased count and motility as well as with sexual dysfunction (impotence, erectile dysfunction and retrograde ejaculation). Prolactin could possibly produce impotence independently from its suppressive effect on testosterone. Stress, many pharmacological substances (e.g. phenothiazines, tricyclic antidepressants, antihypertensives) and hypothyroidism can induce hyperprolactinemia. Treatment of idiopathic hyperprolactinemia consists of dopamine antagonists (e.g. bromocryptine). The literature is controversial about improvement of semen parameters after restoration to a normoprolactinemic state.

1. Ishikawa, H., Kaneko, S., Ohashi, M., Nakagawa, K. and Hata, M. (1993). Retrograde ejaculation accompanying hyperprolactinemia. *Arch. Androl.*, 30(3), 153

2. Laufer, N., Jafee, H. and Margialoth, E. (1981). Effect of bromocryptine treatment on male infertility associated with hyperprolactinemia. *Arch. Androl.*, 6, 343

3. Mancini, A., Guitelman, A. and Levalle, O. (1984). Bromocryptine in the management of infertile men after surgery of prolactin secreting adenomas. *J. Androl.*, 5, 294

Related subjects: bromocryptine, endocrinology, hyperprolactinemia, hypogonadotropic hypogonadism, impotence, prolactin, microadenoma, retrograde ejaculation

HYPERSPERMIA

Consistent production of an increased volume of the ejaculate of more than 6.3 ml (95th percentile). This condition probably interferes negatively with fertility because of dilution of spermatozoa. There is no agreement in the literature about the upper limit of normal seminal fluid volume. Sometimes no value is given at all (World Health Organization, 1993), while at others a value of 6.0–6.5 ml is proposed. In the case of infertility and hyperspermia, therapy with split ejaculate could be indicated.

1. Cooke, S., Tyler, J.P.P. and Driscoll, G.L. (1995). Hyperspermia: the forgotten condition? *Hum. Reprod.*, 10(2), 367

Related subjects: ejaculate — composition, semen analysis — normal values, split ejaculate

HYPOGONADOTROPIC HYPOGONADISM

Morphological or functional disorders of the hypothalamus or the pituitary may lead to disturbance of normal gonadotropin releasing hormone secretion or release, with ensuing decrease in follicle stimulating hormone (FSH) and luteinizing hormone (LH) output or primary disturbances in the FSH and/ or LH secretion. As a result, spermatogenesis is partially or completely arrested. Table 17 lists the most common causes.

1. Beitins, I.Z., Axelrod, L., Ostrea, T., Little, R. and Badger, T.M. (1981). Hypogonadism in a male with an immunologically active, biologically inactive luteinizing hormone: characterization of the abnormal hormone. *J. Clin. Endocrinol. Metab.*, 52, 1143

2. Santen, R.J. (1981). Male hypogonadism. In Yen, S.S.C. and Jaffe, R.B. (eds.) *Reproductive Endocrinology*, 3rd edn. (Philadelphia: W.B. Saunders)

Related subjects: acquired immuno deficiency syndrome, hyperprolactinemia, Kallmann's syndrome, liver disease, medication — negative effects, obesity, radiation, renal disease, spinal cord injury, stress, tuberculosis

HYPO-OSMOTIC SWELLING TEST

If the sperm plasma membrane is intact, as is the case in viable sperm cells, exposure to a hypo-osmotic medium will cause an influx of water in an effort to reach osmotic equilibrium. As a result the sperm tail will swell. The ability of the spermatozoon to swell under hypo-osmotic conditions is a sign that fluid transport across the membrane occurs normally, thus indicating membrane integrity. The literature gives no proof of a solid correlation of this test with fertilizing capacity, thus leaving it as a test of sperm viability.

1. Jeyendran, R.S., van der Ven, H.H. and Zaneveld, L.J. (1992). The hypoosmotic swelling test: an update. *Arch. Androl.*, 29(2), 105

Related subjects: sperm function tests

HYPOSPADIA

This is a congenital abnormality resulting in incomplete development of the anterior urethra. The meatal opening can be located anywhere on the dorsal side of the shaft of the penis, even on the perineum. Several surgical techniques are being employed for correction. Depending on the success of surgical repair, aiming the deposition of semen into the posterior vagina and the possible involvement of other factors affecting sperm quality, intra-cervical (ICI) or intrauterine insemination (IUI) are indicated. The most common anomaly associated with the condition is undescended testis. The inheritance of hypospadia is multifactorial, depending on the associated pathology, and it has an incidence of 0.3–0.8% of all male births.

Table 17 The most common causes of hypogonadotropic hypogonadism in men

Category	Disorder	Comment
Organic process of hypothalamus– pituitary	idiopathic tumors vascular infiltrative	most common in adolescence craniopharyngioma collagen disease, infarction tuberculosis, sarcoidosis, histiocytosis
Hyperprolactinemia		direct inhibition of GnRH release mechanical suppression of hypothalamus or pituitary
Isolated gonadotropin deficiency	complete form – FSH and LH predominant LH deficiency bio-inactive LH production	Kallman's syndrome fertile eunuch (FSH stimulates spermatogenesis) elevated immunoreactive LH and low testosterone found
Genetic syndromes	Prader–Willi Laurence–Moon–Biedl	
Acute or chronic illness	malnutrition stress AIDS obesity medication renal disease liver disease hemochromatosis spinal cord injury	deficient GnRH release inhibited release of GnRH by elevated corticotropin releasing low androgen levels; cause is controversial low LH and testosterone narcotics, glucocorticoids abnormal feedback due to hypothalamic dysfunction malnutrition, enhanced aromatization, increased estrogen negative feedback primary or secondary (thalassemia); iron overload of pituitary low testosterone in more than half of the patients

FSH = follicle stimulating hormone; LH = luteinizing hormone, GnRH = gonadotropin releasing hormone

Hashmat, A.I. and Das, S. (1993). *The Penis*. (Philadelphia: Lea and Febiger)

Related subjects: cryptorchidism, insemination, orchidopexy

HYPOTAURINE

Compound derived from cysteine and as such an (active) precursor of taurine. Both compounds are known to have important anti-oxidative properties.

Related subjects: antioxidants, oxygen reactive species, sperm preparation, taurine

HYPOTHYROIDISM

Hypothyroidism is a rare (0.6%), but well documented form of male infertility. Follicle stimulating hormone and luteinizing hormone are normal, while prolactin and testosterone are often elevated. Semen analysis shows abnormalities in all parameters and sexual dysfunction may be present. Hypothyroidism is estimated to be present in a subclinical form in 3% of the male population.

1. Buitrago, J. and Diez, L. (1987). Serum hormones and seminal parameters in males with thyroid disturbance. *Andrologia*, 19, 37

2. Helfand, M. and Crapo, L. (1990). Screening for thyroid disease. *Ann. Int. Med.*, 112, 840

Related subjects: hyperprolactinemia, sexual dysfunction

HUMAN CHORIONIC GONADOTROPIN (hCG)

A glycoprotein produced by the placenta. It is biologically similar to luteinizing hormone. In hypogonadotropic hypogonadism, hCG is used together with human menopausal gonadotropin (hMG) in men to restore sperm production. The usual schedule is commencement of hCG in a dose of 1500–3000 IU two or three times a week. After 8–12 weeks, follicle stimulating hormone in the form of hMG is added in a dose of 37.5–150 IU two to four times per week. hCG is discontinued when semen parameters come to an acceptable level, since hCG alone can maintain spermatogenesis. The onset of spermatogenesis starts, on average, after 3–6 months, but may be delayed up to 24 months. Treatment success is correlated with the pretreatment testicular volume.

Another indication for hCG in male infertility is in the treatment of cryptorchidism. Here it is sometimes used in an attempt before surgery to correct the malpositioned testes. In these cases hCG can also be used as a test to differentiate between undescended testicles and agonadism and anorchism. Given in in a dose of 1000–2000 IU three times a week, testosterone levels will rise markedly in a case of undescended testes.

1. Santen, R.J. (1991). Male hypogonadism. In Yen, S.S.C. and Jaffe, R.B. (eds.) *Reproductive Endocrinology*. (Philadelphia: W.B.Saunders)

2. Sherins, R. (1984). *Evaluation and Management of Hypogonadotropic Hypogonadism.* (Philadelphia: B.C. Decker)

Related subjects: cryptorchidism, follicle stimulating hormone, human menopausal gonadotropin, hypogonadotropic hypogonadism, medication — treatment

HUMAN IMMUNODEFICIENCY VIRUS (HIV)

Human immunodeficiency virus-1 or human lymphotropic retrovirus-3 (HTLV-3) binds to the CD4 protein of T4 cells (lymphocytes, monocytes). It may stay dormant or cause infection, causing the death of the host cells. In men, T4 cells are most numerous in the epididymis and the prostate. The virus is supposed to migrate into the male genital tract via infected leucocytes and monocytes, since it has been isolated from seminal and prostatic secretions. Its presence in the male genital tract is an important source of spread of the disease. Seropositivity for HIV is associated with other sexually transmitted diseases such as gonorrhea, *Chlamydia*, syphilis and cytomegaly. Once HIV progresses to immunosuppression, acquired immunodeficiency syndrome develops.

1. Kwan, D.J. and Lowe, F.C. (1992). Acquired immunodeficiency syndrome. In Mellinger, B.C. and Smith, A.D. (eds.) Sexually transmitted diseases. *Urol. Clin. N. Am.*, 19(1)

Related subjects: acquired immunodeficiency syndrome

HUMAN MENOPAUSAL GONADOTROPIN (hMG)

A preparation of gonadotropins extracted from urine of perimenopausal women. Usually it is commercially available in a ratio of follicle stimulating hormone to human chorionic gonadotropin hormone of 1:1. Preparations with a different ratio (usually a decreased amount of luteinizing hormone) are also marketed. For treatment of hypogonadotropic hypogonadism and restoration of spermatogenesis see under human chorionic gonadotropin hormone.

Related subjects: follicle stimulating hormone, human chorionic gonadotropin, hypogonadotropic hypogonadism, luteinizing hormone, medication — treatment

I i

IMMOTILE CILIA SYNDROME

This is the alternative name for the ciliary dyskinesis syndrome. These patients present with asthenozoospermia. The reported structural abnormalities of spermatozoa include: inner and/or outer dynein arms or spokes missing, and absent or defective central microtubules. The diagnosis can be made by electron microscopy. These patients have structural abnormalities of their cilia. Ciliated epithelium can be found in nasal passages and sinuses, the middle ear mucosa, pharynx and upper respiratory tract. Although the oviduct has ciliated epithelium, affected females seem to have normal fertility rates. The prevalence of the condition is 1:20 000. It is an autosomal recessive disease.

1. Afzelius, B.A. (1981). Genetical and ultrastructural aspects of the immotile cilia syndrome. *Am. J. Hum. Genet.*, **33**, 852

Related subjects: asthenozoospermia, morphology — normal

IMPOTENCE

Anejaculation due to inability to attain or to sustain a penile erection.

Related subjects: diabetes mellitus, hypergonadotropic hypogonadism, hyperprolactinemia, liver disease, sexual function — drugs, sexual function — terminology

INHIBIN

This is a glycoprotein hormone appearing in two heterodimer forms: inhibin A (α-subunit and βA-subunit) and inhibin B (α-subunit and βB-subunit). Sertoli cells are the major source of synthesis and secretion and inhibin action consists mainly of inhibition of follicle stimulating hormone (FSH) secretion by the pituitary. The biosynthesis of inhibin is stimulated by FSH, growth factors and sex steroid hormones.

1. Veldhuis, J. (1991). The hypothalamic–pituitary–testicular axis. In Yen, S.S.C. and Jaffe, R.B. (eds.) *Reproductice Endocrinology*, 3rd edn. (Philadelphia: W.B. Saunders)

Related subjects: activin, endocrinology, Sertoli cell

INSEMINATION, ARTIFICIAL

The method by which semen is collected from husband or donor and brought into the female genital tract by means other than sexual intercourse:

(1) Intravaginally (IVI);

(2) Intracervically (ICI);

(3) Intrauterine (IUI);

(4) Intrafallopian tube (IFI), or Fallopian tube perfusion (FSP);

(5) Intrafollicular (DIFI); and

(6) Intraperitoneally (DIPI).

Generally, the latter two forms of insemination are considered not to be forms of insemination. A prerequisite to perform insemination is the presence of normal pelvic anatomy (e.g. the presence of at least one patent tube). There are several indications for artificial insemination. These are:

(1) Abnormal male penile anatomy (hypospadia) and/or physiology (e.g. retrograde ejaculation);

(2) Sexual dysfunction;

(3) Poor/absent cervical mucus;

(4) Negative mucus–sperm interaction tests;

(5) Impaired sperm quality;

(6) Immunological, male or female;

(7) Unexplained infertility; and

(8) Time-limited chances for conception.

Only mechanical problems (such as hypospadias with normal semen analysis) and insemination with donor semen are considered to be valid indications for intracervical insemination. A randomized, controlled study in couples with impaired sperm–cervical interaction showed no beneficial effects of intracervical insemination over no treatment. Except for intravaginal and intracervical insemination, the spermatozoa have to be prepared (selected). Placement of unprepared semen into the uterine cavity has disadvantages, such as painful contractions because of the prostaglandin content of seminal fluid and the possible risk of the transfer of micro-organisms beyond the natural cervical mucus barrier. Because yields of progressively motile spermatozoa are unpredictable, the intended sperm preparation technique should be evaluated before the start of the treatment. Apart from the applied technique of insemination and whether and if, how the semen is prepared, results depend also on other factors. The application of ovarian (hyper)stimulation, and the method by which the timing of the insemination is done, are important methodological variations with impact on the outcome. Finally, the indication for insemination is clearly a determinant of pregnancy rates. Normally in intrauterine insemination a maximum volume of 0.5 ml is installed in the uterine cavity. Some studies claim that if the volume is increased to 4 ml and thus at least part of the semen is perfused into the Fallopian tubes, success rates are higher than with low volume treatment. The results of the review of the literature on intrauterine insemination are shown in Table 18.

Table 18   A review of the literature on intrauterine insemination (IUI)

Category	Variable	Pregnancy rate		Comment
Indication for IUI	cervical	mean per cycle: unstimulated clomiphene hMG	 13.8% 16.7% 14.5%	large variation; lack of definition of cervical factor; no controlled studies
	male factor	mean/range/cycle: unstimulated clomiphene hMG	 5.5(0–20)% 6.7(3–12)% 10(3–17)%	lack of uniformity in definition of abnormal semen; different methods of semen preparation
	unexplained infertility	mean per cycle: unstimulated clomiphene hMG	 5.8% 18.8% 18.2%	few controlled studies
	immunological	per cycle: unstimulated clomiphene hMG	 3% 7% 11%	study in patients with female antibodies; other studies not conclusive
Ovarian (hyper) stimulation	clomiphene	per cycle: unstimulated clomiphene	 1.5–4.5% 3–12%	due to IUI or to clomiphene?
	hMG	per cycle: unstimulated hMG	 0–6.7% 7.1–19%	requires close monitoring; no controlled studies of sufficient sample size; risk of ovarian hyperstimulation and multiple pregnancy
Timing of insemination	hCG			controversy about optimal time
	urinary LH peak			more physiological
Number of inseminations	one two	8–11%/cycle 14–52%/cycle		controversial results in different studies
Number of cycles				most studies report that the majority of pregnancies are obtained within four treatment cycles

hMG = human menopausal gonadotropin; hCG = human chorionic gonadotropin; LH = luteinizing hormone

1. Dodson, W.C. and Haney, A.F. (1981). Controlled ovarian hyperstimulation and intrauterine insemination for treatment of infertility. *Fertil. Steril.*, 55(3), 457

2. Friedman, A.J., Juneau-Norcross, M., Sedensky, B., Andrews, N., Dorfman, J. and Cramer, D.W. (1991). Life table analysis of intrauterine insemination pregnancy rates for couples with cervical factor, male factor, and idiopathic infertility. *Fertil. Steril.*, 55(5), 1005

3. Glazener, C.M.A., Coulson, C. and Lambert, P.A. (1987). The value of artificial insemination with husband's semen in infertility due to failure of postcoital sperm–mucus penetration – controlled trial of treatment. *Br. J. Obstet. Gynaecol.*, 94, 774

4. Kahn, J.A., Sunde, A., Koskemies, A., von During, V., Sordal, T., Christensen, F. and Molne, K. (1993). Fallopian tube sperm perfusion (FSP) versus intra-uterine insemination (IUI) in the treatment of unexplained infertility: a prospective randomized study. *Hum. Reprod.*, 8(6), 890

5. Margialoth, E.J., Sauter, E. and Bronson, R.A. (1988). Intrauterine insemination as treatment for antisperm antibodies in the female. *Fertil. Steril.*, 50, 441

6. Martinez, A.R., Bernardus, R.E., Vermeiden, J.P.W. and Schoemaker, J. (1993). Basic questions on intrauterine insemination: an update. *Obstet. Gynecol. Surv.*, 48(12), 811

7. Nulsen, J.C., Walsh, S., Dumez, S. and Metzger, D.A. (1993). A randomized and longitudinal study of human menopausal gonadotropin with intrauterine insemination in the treatment of infertility. *Obstet. Gynecol.*, 82, 780

8. Ransom, M.X., Blotner, M.B., Bohrer, M., Corsan, G. and Kemmann, G. (1994). Does increasing frequency of intrauterine insemination improve pregnancy rates significanly during superovulation cycles? *Fertil. Steril.*, 61(2), 303

9. Silverberg, K.M., Johnson, J.V., Olive, D.L., Burns, W.N. and Schenken, R.S. (1992). A prospective randomized trial comparing two different intrauterine insemination regimens in controlled ovarian hyperstimulation cycles. *Fertil. Steril.*, 57, 357

Related subjects: assisted reproduction, direct intrafollicular insemination, direct intraperitoneal insemination, sperm preparation

INTRACYTOPLASMIC SPERM INJECTION (ICSI)

An advanced reproductive technique in which a single spermatozoon is aspirated into a micropipette and injected into the oocyte. Any type of sperm with haploid chromosome content can be injected. Previous capacitation and acrosome reaction appear to be unnecessary. Pricking the oocyte and infusion of the injection medium and the spermatozoon seems to activate the oocyte. Fertilization rates of around 60% are reported. These fertilization rates are independent of semen parameters and the way the semen is collected. As the method bypasses all the biological selectivity, some concern about chromosomal abnormality is valid. So far, these concerns have not materialized in the children born after *in vitro* fertilization–ICSI. Present indications include severe male factor and unexplained fertilization failure.

1. Palermo, G., Joris, H., Devroey, P. and van Steirteghem, A.C. (1992). Pregnancies after intracytoplasmic sperm injection of a single spermatozoon into an oocyte. *Lancet*, 340, 17

2. Palermo, G.D., Cohen, J., Alikani, M., Adler, A. and Rosenwaks, Z. (1995). Intracytoplasmic sperm injection: a novel treatment for all forms of male factor infertility. *Fertil. Steril.*, **63**(6), 1231

3. van Steirteghem, A.C., Zsolt, N., Liu, J., Joris, H., Bonduelle, M. and Devroey, P. (1993). Assisted fertilization by subzonal insemination and intracytoplasmic sperm injection. *J. Assist. Reprod. Genet.*, **10**, 184

Related subjects: assisted reproduction, *in vitro* fertilization, micromanipulation

IN VITRO FERTILIZATION (IVF)

The assisted reproductive technique in which the oocyte and a number of prepared spermatozoa are brought together in culture medium and thereafter incubated in order to achieve fertilization. Originally, the method was developed for, and applied to, patients with irreversible tubal obstruction. At present, impaired semen quality is a common indication for IVF, but success rates generally are less than in patients with normal semen parameters. The fertilization rate decreases directly with the total number of motile spermatozoa available for insemination. Only if an adequate number of motile spermatozoa after semen preparation cannot be obtained, micromanipulation, and more specifically intraytoplasmic sperm injection, should be considered primarily. Generally the required number of motile spermatozoa thought to be necessary for standard IVF is reported as 50 000 per oocyte, 100 000 per culture dish or 500 000 total.

1. Ben-Chetrit, A., Senoz, S., Greenblatt, E.M. and Casper, R.F. (1992). *In-vitro* fertilization outcome in the presence of severe male factor infertility. *Fertil. Steril.*, **63**(5), 1032

2. Palermo, G.D., Cohen, J., Alikani, M., Adler, A. and Rosenwaks, Z. (1995). Intracytoplasmic sperm injection: a novel treatment for all forms of male factor infertility. *Fertil. Steril.*, **63**(6):1231

Related subjects: assisted reproduction, micromanipulation, sperm preparation

K*k*

KALLIKREIN

This is a proteinase enzyme which acts on kininogen to produce kinin which is the biologically active polypeptide stimulating vascular permeability, blood flow to the testis and glucose transport. Kallikrein is therefore postulated to enhance sperm metabolism, increase testicular blood flow and improve the Sertoli cell function, resulting in better sperm motility. Meta-analysis of oral kallikrein showed somewhat higher pregnancy rates than placebo in oligozoospermic patients, although the quality of the studies was poor. Treatment of spermatozoa with kallikrein *in vitro* showed significant improvement in sperm density, motility and forward progression.

1. Gilbaugh, J.H. and Lipshultz, L.I. (1994). Non-surgical treatment of male infertility. *Urol. Clin. N. Am.*, **21**(3)

2. Micic, S., Tulic, C. and Dotlic, R. (1990). Kallikrein therapy of infertile men with varicocele and impaired sperm motility. *Andrologia*, **22**, 179

3. O'Donovan, P., Vandekerchhove, P., Lilford, R. and Hughes, E. (1993). Treatment of male infertility. Is it effective? Review and meta analysis of published randomized controlled trials. *Hum. Reprod.*, **8**, 1209

Related subjects: medication – treatment

KALLMANN'S SYNDROME

A syndrome consisting of isolated gonadotropin deficiency with otherwise intact pituitary function. The degree of gonadotropin deficiency may vary. In the complete form both follicle stimulating hormone (FSH) and luteinizing hormone levels are low. With partial deficiency FSH secretion predominates. The condition is associated with hypo- or aplasia of the olfactory tract and bulbs. It is associated with hypo- or anosmia and sometimes with cryptorchidism and congenital defects involving midline facial and head structures such as cleft lip or palate. Males usually present with delayed onset of puberty, micropenis and cryptorchidism. Initiation of spermatogenesis requires gonadotropin releasing hormone or gonadotropins administration. The incidence reported varies from 1 in 10 000 to 1 in 60 000. It has multiple inheritance patterns both X-linked and autosomal, the most common being the X-linked recessive type (KALIG-1 gene).

1. Bick, D., Franco, B. and Sherins, R.J. (1992). Iatrogenic deletion of the KALIG-1 gene in Kallmann's syndrome. *N. Engl. J. Med.*, **326**, 1752

2. Sigman, M. and Howards, S.S. (1992). Male infertility. In Walsh, P.C., Retik, A.B. and Stamey, T.A. (eds.) *Campbell's Urology*, vol. 2. (Philadelphia: W.B. Saunders)

Related subjects: genetics, hypogonadotropic hypogonadism, medication — treatment

KARTAGENER'S SYNDROME

A syndrome, first described in 1933 by Kartagener consisting of situs inversus, bronchiectasis and chronic sinusitis. Fifty percent of the patients with immotile cilia syndrome have features of Kartagener's syndrome. The inheritance is autosomal recessive and its prevalence is 1:40 000.

1. Burn, J. (1991). Disturbance of morphological laterality in humans (review). *Ciba Foundation Symposium*, 162, 282

Related subjects: ciliary dyskenesis, immotile cilia syndrome

KLINEFELTER'S SYNDROME

This is a chromosomal disorder with a 47 XXY pattern. These men present with azoospermia, gynecomasty and tall stature. Follicle stimulating hormone and luteinizing hormone levels are increased, but testosterone decreased in 50% of cases. The testes are atrophic, firm and less than 2 cm. Testicular biopsy shows hyalinized tubules, relative Leydig cell hyperplasia and absence of spermatogenesis. In the mosaic forms there is an increased incidence of cryptorchidism. Up to 10% are mosaics, which makes this the most common male developmental defect: 1 in 500 men are affected. Fertility is documented in mosaic forms.

1. Griffin, J.E. and Wilson, J.D. (1992). Disorders of sexual differentiation. In Walsh, P.C., Retik, A. and Stamey, T.A. (eds.) *Campbell's Urology*, Vol. 2. (Philadelphia: W.B. Saunders)

2. Harari, O., Gronow, M., Bourne, H., Johnston, I. and Baker, G. (1992). High fertilization rate with intracytoplasmatic sperm injection in mosaic Klinefelter's syndrome. *Fertil. Steril.*, 63(1), 183

3. Terzol, G., Lalatta, F., Lobbiani, A., Simoni, G. and Colluci, G. (1992). Fertility in 47XXY patient: assesment of biological paternity by deoxyribonucleic acid fingerprinting. *Fertil. Steril.*, 58, 821,

Related subjects: azoospermia, chromosomal abnormalities, cryptorchidism, hypergonadotropic hypogonadism

KREMER TEST

In vitro test for sperm migration into cervical mucus. A capillary tube with preovulatory cervical mucus is placed in a reservoir of spermatozoa. The depth of sperm penetration is evaluated microscopically. The test is used when the postcoital test is difficult to evaluate. The outcome of the test is strongly influenced by the number of progressive motile at the sperm–mucus interface.

1. Kremer, J. (1965). A simple sperm penetration test. *Int. J. Fertil.*, **10**, 209

2. Insler, V. and Bettendorf, G.(eds.) (1977). *The Uterine Cervix in Reproduction*. (Stuttgart: Georg Thieme)

Related subjects: Kurzrok–Miller test, postcoital test, sperm–cervical mucus contact test, sperm function test

KURZROK–MILLER TEST

In vitro test for sperm migration into cervical mucus. A drop of cervical mucus is removed at midcycle and opposed against a drop of semen and placed under a coverslide. The depth of sperm penetration is then evaluated. The test is largely replaced by the Kremer test and/or bovine mucus test because of difficulties in reproducibility.

1. Kurzrok, R. and Miller, E.G. (1928). Biochemical studies of human semen and its relation to mucus of the cervix uteri. *Am. J. Obstet. Gynecol.*, **15**, 56

2. Insler, V. and Bettendorf, G. (eds.) (1977). *The Uterine Cervix in Reproduction*. (Stuttgart: Georg Thieme)

Related subjects: Kremer test, postcoital test, sperm–cervical mucus contact test, sperm function test

L*l*

LECTINS

Lectins are proteins or glycoproteins which cause cell agglutination and/or precipitate complex carbohydrates. Lectins have been isolated from many natural sources (seeds, plant roots and bark, fungi, bacteria, body fluids, cell membranes, etc.). Their specific role in nature has not been fully elucidated, but their use in the field of andrology is widespread. The most common lectins used in sperm function testing are *Pisum sativum* (PSA), concanavalin A (ConA) and *Arachis hypogaea* (PNA). Each lectin is specific for a certain sugar residue. Specifically, lectins have been used to detect and monitor the acrosome reaction of human spermatozoa: the binding of different lectins to the sperm cell membranes may be assessed cytochemically using fluorescent dyes, biotin or colloidal gold-labelled lectins. In this way, a crude determination of the acrosomal status of the spermatozoa may be performed: however, flow cytometric analysis, coupled with monoclonal antibody binding studies, has now superceded many of the early assays.

1. Carver-Ward, J.A., Jaroudi, K.A., Einspenner, M., Parhar, R.S., Al-Sedairy, S.T. and Sheth, K.V. (1994). Pentoxifylline potentiates ionophore (A23187) mediated acrosome reaction in human sperm: flow cytometric analysis using CD46 antibody. *Hum. Reprod.*, 9(1), 71

2. D'Cruz, O.J., Haas, G.G. Jr and Lambert, H. (1993). Heterogeneity of human sperm surface antigens identified by indirect immunoprecipitation of antisperm antibody bound to biotinylated sperm. *J. Immunol.*, 151(2), 1062

3. Mladenovic, I., Hajdukovic, L., Genbacev, O., Cuperlovic, M. and Movsesijan, M. (1993). Lectin binding a a biological test *in vitro* for the prediction of functional activity of human spermatozoa. *Hum. Reprod.*, 8(2), 258

Related subjects: acrosome reaction — test, flow cytometry

LEUKOCYTOSPERMIA

According to the World Health Organization's definition more than 1 million leukocytes/ml of semen are considered to be abnormal. Sometimes it is difficult to distinguish leukocytes from immature germ cells using conventional staining. Monoclonal antibodies specific for leukocytes are more effective in this regard. The condition is correlated with reduced count, decreased motility, abnormal morphology, negative effect on the postcoital test and *in vitro* mucus penetration. It is also a prognostic factor for fertilization failure *in vitro*. The etiology of the condition is often not clear.

It can be associated with bacterial or viral infection, although 80% of leukocytospermic samples are microbiologically negative. Association also exists with environmental factors such as cigarette smoking, abnormal spermatogenesis, abstinence and clinical situations like varicocele. Mechanisms thought to be involved are release of cytokines (interferon-γ, TNF-α), reactive nitrogen intermediates and reactive oxygen species (see also table STD). White blood cells in semen can carry pathogens like HIV, cytomegaly virus and *Chlamydia* and thus might be an important factor in transmission of such diseases.

1. Anderson, D.J. (1995). Should male infertility patients be tested for leukocytospermia? *Fertil. Steril.* 63(2), 246
2. Eggert-Kruse, W., Bellmann, A., Rohr, G., Tilgen, W. and Runnebaum, B. (1992). Differentiation of round cells in semen by means of monoclonal antibodies and relationship with male infertility. *Fertil. Steril.*, 58, 1046
3. Wolff, H. (1995). The biologic significance of white blood cells in semen. *Fertil. Steril.*, 63(6), 114
4. World Health Organization (1992). *WHO Semen Manual for the Examination of Human Semen and Cervical Mucus.* (Cambridge: Cambridge University Press)

Related subjects: bacterial infection, cigarette smoking, culture — semen, oxygen — reactive species, semen analysis — normal values, sexually transmitted diseases

LEYDIG CELL

The Leydig cells or interstitial cells are located exterior to the seminiferous tubules within the connective tissue stroma of the testis (see Figure 13). Differentiation takes place in the seventh week of pregnancy, probably under the influence of human chorionic gonadotropin and from then onwards they start synthesizing and secreting testosterone. Reactivation starts at puberty, but can be initiated any time before by exposure to gonadotropins. Leydig cells are the major source of testosterone in males, since they secrete 95% of the circulating testosterone. They also secrete activin which has a positive effect on follicle stimulating hormone secretion.

1. Veldhuis, J. (1991). The hypothalamic–pituitary–testicular axis. In Yen, S.S.C. and Jaffe, R. B. (ed.) *Reproductive Endocrinology*, 3rd edn. (Philadelphia: W.B.Saunders)

Related subjects: endocrinology, Sertoli cell, testosterone

LIVER DISEASE, CIRRHOSIS

The effects of liver disease occur independently of the etiology (virus or direct toxic effect of alcohol). Common findings are gynecomastia, testicular atrophy and impotence. Patients with both hypogonadotropic and hypergonadotropic states may be seen. The level of testosterone correlates with the severity of the disease. In the hypogonadotropic group, malnutrition and increased aromatization of testosterone to estradiol may possibly suppress

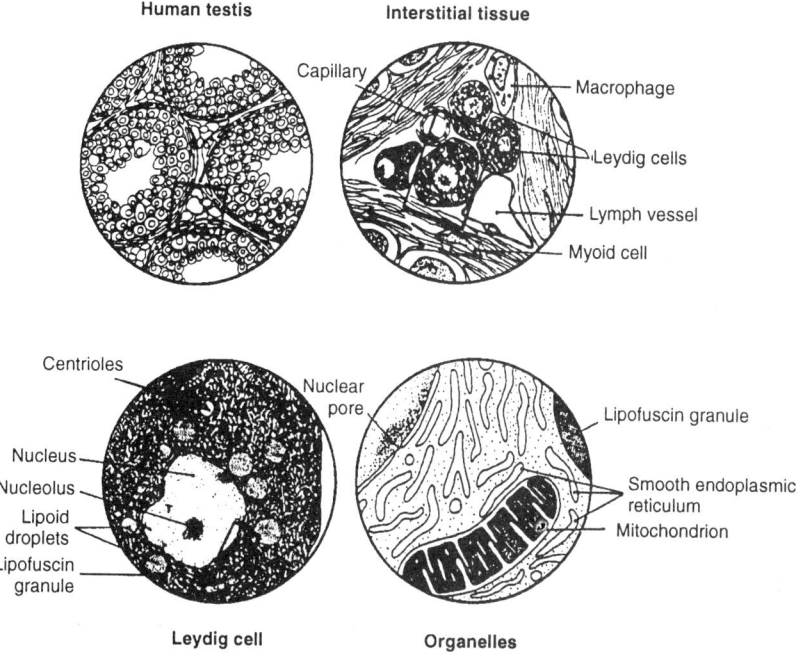

Figure 13 Location and fine structure of Leydig cells. Leydig cells occur in clusters in the interstitial tissue between the seminiferous tubules (upper left). Interstitial tissue (upper right) contains macrophages and fibroblasts as well as capillaries and lymph vessels. Seminiferous tubules are surrounded by a boundary of myoid cells. The most abundant organelle within the cytoplasm of the Leydig cell is the smooth endoplasmic reticulum (lower left). Some of the organelles are seen in greater detail in a selected area of cytoplasm (lower right). (Adapted from Christensen, A. K.: Leydig cells. In Greep, R. O. and Ashwood, E. B. (eds): *Handbook of Physiology*, Section 7. Endocrinology. Baltimore, The William & Wilkins Co., 1975. Copyright 1975. The American Physiological Society, Bethesda, Md.)

follicle stimulating hormone and luteinizing hormone levels. Hypergonadotropic patients have a primary testicular dysfunction.

1. De Besi, L., Zuchetta, P. and Zotti, S. (1989). Sex hormones and sex hormone binding globulin in males with compensated and decompensated cirrhosis of the liver. *Acta Endocrinol.*, **120**, 271

2. Gluud, C. and the Copenhagen Study Group for Liver Disesases (1987). Serum testosterone concentrations in men with alcoholic cirrhosis: background for variation. *Metabolism*, **45**, 145

Related subjects: alcohol, hypogonadotropic hypogonadism, hypergonadotropic hypogonadism, impotence, nutritional deficiencies

LUTEINIZING HORMONE (LH)

LH is a glycoprotein hormone with two subunits: one α- and one LH β-subunit. Production is in the pars distalis of the anterior pituitary. It is secreted in a pulsatile way with a frequency of 60–90 minutes. LH regulates testosterone biosynthesis in the Leydig cells. After initiation of spermatogenesis LH alone is capable to maintain this process. LH therapy is indicated in the restoration of spermatogenesis in hypogonadotropic hypogonadism and in the medical treatment of cryptorchidism. Usually it is administered in the form of human chorionic gonadotropin which exhibits LH-like activity. In case of the restoration of spermatogenesis it is often used in combination with follicle stimulating hormone. See also under human chorionic gonadotropin.

1. Veldhuis, J. (1991). The hypothalamic–pituitary–testicular axis. In Yen, S.S.C. and Jaffe, R.B. (eds.) *Reproductive Endocrinology*, 3rd edn. (Philadelphia: W.B. Saunders)

Related subjects: follicle stimulating hormone, human chorionic gonadotropin, hypogonadotropic hypogonadism, medication — treatment

LUTEINIZING HORMONE RELEASING HORMONE

See gonadotropin releasing hormone.

M*m*

MAGNETIC RESONANCE IMAGING (MRI)

Magnetic resonance imaging is a non-ionizing technique providing cross-sectional images. The basic principle is the fact that in a strong external magnetic field, nuclei with an even number of neutrons or protons will align within the external field. In the human body with its abundance of hydrogen, MRI is performed with protons. Application of a specific radiofrequency, directly related to the strength of the magnetic field, will cause dealignment, removal of the radiofrequency pulse gradually restores realignment with the external field. The emitted energy during realignment is the signal employed to form the image. Magnetic resonance imaging provides high quality soft tissue contrast resolution. So far, no immediate or delayed biological or genetic defects have been identified, although validation over a longer follow-up period is necessary. Since MRI gives excellent images of anatomic structures within the pelvis, it can provide detailed information about abnormalities related to male fertility. The pathology listed in Table 19 related to male infertility can be visualized by MRI as a first modality or be employed if other imaging techniques provide no conclusive information.

Table 19 The uses of magnetic resonance imaging (MRI) in male infertility

	Pathology	First choice	Second choice
Testis	congenital: anorchia; cryptorchidism	MRI	
	torsion	color Doppler flow	
	varicocele	ultrasound	MRI
	epididymitis	ultrasound	MRI
Seminal vesicle	congenital: agenesis; hypoplasia	ultrasound	MRI
	infection	ultrasound	MRI
Prostate	cyst	ultrasound	MRI
	infection	ultrasound	computerized tomography (CT) scanning

1. Hricak, H. and Carrington, B.M. (1991). *MRI of the Pelvis.* (London: Martin Dunitz Ltd)

Related subjects: ultrasonography

MEDICATION, TREATMENT OF MALE INFERTILITY (Table 20)

Review of the literature dealing with medical treatment of abnormal semen parameters and male infertility shows that many of these treatments are either based upon theoretical grounds without ever being tested in a well designed study or are subjected to studies not meeting standard requirements.

1. Carreras, A. and Mendoza, C. (1990). Zinc levels in seminal plasma of fertile and infertile men. *Andrologia*, 22(3), 279

2. Clark, R. and Sherins, R. (1989). Clinical trial of testolactone for treatment of idiopathic male infertility. *J. Androl.*, 10, 240

3. Lanzafame, F., Chapman, M.G., Guglielmino, A., Gearon, C.M. and Forman, R.G. (1994). Pharmacological stimulation of sperm motility. *Hum. Reprod.*, 9(2), 192

4. O'Donovan, P.A., Vandekerckhove, P., Lilford, R.J. and Hughes, E. (1993). Treatment of male infertility: is it effective? Review and meta-analyses of published randomized controlled trials. *Hum. Reprod.*, 8, 1209

5. Santen, R.J. (1991). Male hypogonadism. In Yen, S.S.C. and Jaffe, R.B. (eds.) *Reproductive Endocrinology.* (Philadelphia: W.B. Saunders)

6. Schill, W.B., Schneider, J. and Ring, J. (1996). The use of ketotifen, a mast cell blocker, for treatment of oligo- and asthenozoospermia. *Andrologia*, 18(57), 573

7. Schopohl, J., Mehltretter, G. and Zumbusch, R.V. (1991). Comparison of gonadotropin-releasing hormone and gonadotropin therapy in male patients with idiopathic hypogonadotropic hypogonadism. *Fertil. Steril.*, 56, 1143

8. Tesarik, J. and Mendoza, C. (1993). Sperm treatment with pentoxifylline improves the fertilizing ability in patients with acrosome reaction insufficiency. *Fertil. Steril.*, 60, 141

9. Tournaye, H., van Steirteghem, A.C. and Devroey, P. (1994). Pentoxifylline in idiopathic male-factor infertility: a review of its therapeutic efficacy after oral administration. *Hum. Reprod.*, 9(6), 996

10. Yovich, J.L. (1993). Pentoxifylline: actions and applications in assisted reproduction. *Hum. Reprod.*, 8(11), 1786

Related subjects: androgen therapy, anti-oxidants, antisperm antibodies, bacterial infection, hypogonadotropic hypogonadism, hyperprolactinemia, prostatitis, retrograde ejaculation, taurine

MEDICATION WITH NEGATIVE EFFECT ON SPERMATOGENESIS (Table 21)

In this overview antibiotics, drugs and cytostatics are not included. They are described under a separate heading.

1. Olin, B.R. (ed.) (1994). *Drug, Facts and Comparisons.* (St.Louis: Facts and Comparison Inc.)

2. Duke, M.N.G. (ed.) (1988). *Meyler's Side Effects on Drugs*, 11th edition. (Amsterdam: Elsevier)

Related subjects: antibiotics — negative effects, drug abuse, cytostatics

Table 20   The medical treatment of male infertility

Group	Type	Indication	Remarks
GnRH		hypogonadotropic hypogonadism	pulsatile i.v. or s.c. 5–30 µg/2 hrs
FSH	hMG, pure FSH	hypogonadotropic hypogonadism	37.5–150 IU 1–3 times a week
LH	hCG	hypogonadotropic hypogonadism (+hMG) cryptorchidism	1000–3000 IU 1–3 times a week
Androgens	testosterone enanthate testosterone cypionate testosterone undecanoate fluoxymesterone methyltestosterone	substitution in case of hypogonadism; aim at blood level of 300–1200 ng/dl	testosterone enanthate and cypionate 100–300 mg/ 1–3 weeks; testosterone undecanoate 200 mg; fluoxymesterone 5–10 mg o.d.; methyl-testosterone 25 mg
Antiestrogens	clomiphene, tamoxifen	hypo- or normogonado-tropic, abnormal sperm analysis	effect not proven
Aromatase inhibitor	testolactone	idiopathic oligozoospermia	effect not proven
Dopamine agonists	bromocriptine	hyperprolactinemia	effect on sexual dysfunction is clear; on sperm parameters controversial
Antibiotics	tetradoxycycline, co-trimoxazole, quinolones	acute or chronic infection of male sexual glands	
Anti-phlogistics	prostaglandin synthetase; inhibitors, aspirin	adjunct to antibiotics in epididymitis and orchitis	increased number of mast cells to be proven by
Mast cell blockers	ketotifen	epididymitis, orchitis	biopsy; effect not proven
Immuno-suppression	corticosteroids	antisperm antibodies	increased fertility not proven
Methyl-xanthines (cyclic AMP phospho-diesterase inhibitors)	caffeine, pentoxifylline; theophylline	low motility	caffeine application *in vitro* conflicting results in literature; pentoxifylline not proven effective *per os,* maybe effective in certain patients when applied *in vitro*
Motility stimulator	2-deoxyadenosine; kallkrein	low motility	2-deoxy probably effective *in vitro;* effects of kallikrein controversial
Mineral substitution	zinc	zinc deficiencies (renal, liver)	proven effect only in systemic zinc deficiency
Anti-oxidants	vitamin E; vitamin C	antagonizing of negative effects of reactive oxygen species (e.g. during sperm preparation, in leukocytospermia or in smoking)	effect not proven *per os* addition of antoxidants to culture medium seems beneficial
α-Sympatho-mimetics anticholinergics	mitrodine, imipramine; brompheniramine	retrogade ejaculation; emission failure	

GnRH = gonadotropin releasing hormone, FSH = follicle stimulating hormone, LH = luteinizing hormone, hMG = human menopausal gonadptropin, i.v. = intravenous, s.c. = subcutaneous

Table 21 Medication with a negative effect on spermatogenesis

Drug	Action indication	Effect of semen	Remarks
Cimetidine	histamine H2 antagonist; anti-ulcer agent	reduced sperm count	also impotence and gynecomastia
Colchicine	antimitotic agent; gout	azoospermia	reversible
Corticosteroids	anti-inflammatory; immunosuppressive	reduced sperm count and motility	
Cyproterone acetate	anti-androgen; sexual deviations in male, precocious puberty	reduced spermatogenesis; decreased motility	reversible
Danazol	antigonadotropin; hereditary angio-edema	reduced spermatogenesis; testicular atrophy	short-term use reversible
Finasteride	5α-reductase inhibitor; symptomatic benign prostatic hyperplasia	reduced spermatogenesis	
Gossypol	phenolic compound of cotton plant species; antifertility drug	low motility; azoospermia	reversible?
Halothane	inhalation anesthetic	motility decrease	
Ketoconazole	imidazole broad spectrum antifungal agent	depressed spermatogenesis	low testosterone
Local anesthetics		decreased motility	
Methadone	morphine-like narcotic analgesic; treatment of narcotic addiction	low count and motility; abnormal morphology	reversible
Neuroleptics	several phenothiazines and butyrophenones	oligospermia; polyspermia; necrospermia; decreased motility	reversible
Niridazole	treatment of schistosomiasis	reduced spermatogenesis	reversible
Phenytoin	anticonvulsant	decreased motility; normal FSH, LH, T	
Quinine and derivatives	chloroquine resistant falciparum malaria	decreased motility	reversible
Spironolactone	aldosterone antagonist, antiandrogenic; hyperaldosteronism, hypertension	oligospermia	also gynecomastia

FSH = follicle stimulating hormone, LH = luteinizing hormone, T = testosterone

MICROADENOMA

A microadenoma or prolactinoma refers to a prolactin secreting tumor of the pituitary (hyperplasia) of less than 1 cm diameter located in the sella turcica. The majority of these lesions do not change if the prolactin levels are less than 100 ng/ml.

1. Mancini, A., Guitelman, A. and Levalle, O. (1984). Bromocriptine in the management of infertile men after surgery of prolactin secreting adenomas. *J. Androl.*, 5, 294

Related subjects: bromocriptine, hyperprolactinemia, prolactin

MICROMANIPULATION, GAMETES

Micromanipulation involves microscopic handling of cells with specific instruments (e.g. holding and injection pipettes). Studies reporting injection of spermatozoa directly into the oocyte have been published since 1962. The first study involving human spermatozoa (into hamster oocytes) is from 1976. This early work showed that interactions required for spermatozoa to penetrate the oocyte could be bypassed by direct injection into the oocyte. The different methods commonly used are:

(1) ICSI, intracytoplasmic sperm injection;

(2) SUZI, subzonal insemination;

(3) PZD, partial zona dissection; and

(4) ZD, zona drilling.

1. Hiramoto, Y. (1962). Microinjection of the live spermatozoa into sea urchin eggs. *Exp. Cell Res.*, 27, 416
2. Malter, H.E. and Cohen, J. (1989). Blastocyst formation and hatching *in vitro* following zona drilling of mouse human embryos. *Gamete Res.*, 24, 835
3. van Steirteghem, A.C., Zsolt, N., Liu, J., Joris, H., Bonduelle, M. and Devroey, P. (1993). Assisted fertilization by subzonal insemination and intracytoplasmic sperm injection. *J. Assist. Reprod. Genet.*, 10, 184
4. Uehara, T. and Yanagimachi, R. (1976). Microsurgical injection of spermatozoa into hamster eggs with subsequent transformation of sperm nuclei into male pronuclei. *Biol. Reprod.*, 15, 467

Related subjects: assisted reproduction, intracytoplasmic sperm injection, *in vitro* fertilization, partial zona dissection, subzonal inemination, zona drilling

MICROSCOPY

The compound microscope, which can be applied with or without phase contrast, is the most basic microscope. Compound microscopes enable lower power resolution of spermatozoa (i.e. up to × 400), but they are valuable for rapid identification of major sperm defects (see Table 22). The use of various objectives allows examination of different sperm properties, especially when

Table 22   The use of microsurgery in male infertility

Type microscope	Eye-piece magnification	Objectives	Extras
Compound	10×	20×: motility 40×: SMPA, PCT 100×: morphology. For stained and unstained spermatozoa	phase contrast fluorescence

Inverted	10×	20×, 40×, 100×
		motility assessment in the
		  motility assay and in IVF
		for unstained motile sperma-
		  tozoa. Not recommended
		  for morphology
		also used in micromanipulation
		  procedures	

SMPA = sperm mucus penetration assay, PCT = postcoital test, IVF = *in vitro* fertilization

combined with bright field/dark field in a phase contrast mode. Phase contrast microscopy is an optical system that converts normally invisible phase variations into visible variations in light intensity or contrast. It therefore allows observations on living cells. Staining of the preparation also enhances the microscopic capabilities. Conversely, inverted microscopes are generally used only for low power evaluation of sperm motility.

More complex is the use of fluorescent microscopy, which enables observation of the specimen using the light transmitted or reflected by it. When coupled with fluorescent markers, they enable identification of sperm nuclear and membrane status (i.e. acrosomal integrity). The more recent additions to the market combine phase contrast and fluorescence capabilities within the same model. Most complex and best for evaluation of sperm morphology is TEM (transmission electron microscopy) and SEM (scanning electron microscopy). Electron microscopy uses a magnifying system of beams of electrons focused in a vacuum by a series of magnetic lenses. It enables high magnification and resolution of spermatozoa in order to evaluate surface (SEM) and sectional (TEM) morphology. Scanning electron microscopy enables visualization of the sperm surface, which is mainly valuable for research purposes. Transmission electron microscopy can identify numerous structural defects.

Phase contrast is usually of the Normarski interference contrast type – the limitation of which is that image resolution is poor when used in conjunction with plastics. Therefore, Hoffmann modulation contrast is preferable for micromanipulation unless only glass slides are utilized.

1. Zamboni, L. (1992). Sperm structure and its relevance to infertility. An electron microscopic study. *Arch. Pathol. Lab. Med.*, 116(4), 325–44

Related subjects: morphology — abnormal and normal

MICROSURGERY

Surgical technique employing especially designed instruments, small caliber non-reactive suture materials and minimal tissue handling in order to avoid bleeding, inflammatory reaction and necrosis. An essential part is formed by optical magnification aids such as magnifying spectacles (loupes) and surgical microscopes. Indications for microsurgery for male infertility include vasovasostomy, vaso-epididymostomy, alloplastic and autogenous spermatocele and epididymal sperm aspiration.

1. Gilbert, B.R. (1995). Microsurgical equipment and instrumentation. In Goldstein, M. (ed.) *Surgery for Male Infertility.* (Philadelphia: W.B.Saunders)

Related subjects: micro-epididymal sperm aspiration, vaso-epididymostomy, vasovasostomy, vasectomy reversal

MICROSURGICAL EPIDIDYMAL SPERM ASPIRATION (MESA)

Since 1984 operative sperm aspiration from the epididymis was combined with *in vitro* fertilization in patients with obstructed or congenital absent vas deferens and with certain ejaculatory dysfunctions. The first pregnancy was reported in 1990. Improvement of the pregnancy rates was realized by the introduction of micromanipulation (subzonal insemination and later intracytoplasmic sperm injection) of the obtained sperm. In addition, micropuncture of the epididymis employing very small needles and thus avoiding exposure of the spermatozoa to blood has favoured the results: pregnancy rates of 30%/cycle are now reported. The group of patients with congenital obstruction (congenital absence vas deferens) seems to have a better pregnancy rate than those with secondary obstruction. Possibly, the maturation of epididymal spermatozoa, especially from the more proximal parts, can be improved by treatment with phosphodiesterase inhibitors like pentoxifylline or phosphatidylcholine. Even freezing and thawing of the spermatozoa obtained at the procedure results in very good fertilization and pregnancy rates. Therefore, to avoid further scrotal surgery, freezing of remaining spermatozoa after MESA seems imperative.

1. Belker, A.M., Sherins, R.J., Bustillo, M. and Calvo, M. (1994). Pregnancy with microsurgical vas aspiration from a patient with neurologic ejaculatory dysfunction. *J. Androl.*, 15, 6S

2. Chen, C.S., Chu, S.H., Soong, Y.K. and Lai, Y.M. (1995). Epididymal sperm aspiration with assisted reproductive techniques: difference between congenital and acquired obstructive azoospermia. *Hum. Reprod.*, 10(5), 1104

3. Devroey, P., Silber, S., Nagy, Z., Liu, J., Tournaye, H., Joris, H., Verheyen, G. and van Steirteghem, A. (1995). Ongoing pregnancies and birth after intracytoplasmic sperm injection with frozen-thawed epididymal spermatozoa. *Hum. Reprod.*, 10(4), 903

4. Haidl, G., Badura, B. and Schill, W.B. (1994). Function of human epididymal spermatozoa. *J. Androl.*, 15, 23S

5. Schlegel, P.N., Berkeley, A.S. and Goldstein, M. (1994). Epididymal micropuncture with *in vitro* fertilization and oocyte micromanipulation for the treatment of unreconstructable obstructive azoospermia. *Fertil. Steril.,.* 61, 895

Related subjects: azoospermia, congenital absence vas deferens, cystic fibrosis, micromanipulation, percutaneous epididymal sperm aspiration, testicular sperm aspiration

MORPHOLOGY, ABNORMAL

One main problem of defining normal and abnormal sperm morphology is the unknown fertilizing potential of sperm cells deviating more and more from a modal normal spermatozoon. Another is the enormous variation in abnormal spermatozoa. Many different systems in the past have tried to deal with both aspects. The World Health Organization has developed a system which tries to incorporate the best of all previous classifications. It must be mentioned that very often morphologically abnormal spermatozoa possess multiple defects. For this purpose, in the past, a so-called multiple anomalies index was developed, which proved to be a reliable predictor of fertility. This teratozoospermia index represents the average number of defects per abnormal spermatozoon and ranges from 1.0 to 4.0. All borderline spermatozoa are to be considered abnormal. Some of the most commonly seen abnormalities are listed in Table 23 and shown in Figures 14 to 23).

Table 23   The different types of sperm abnormality

Portion of sperm	Defect
Head	large, small, tapering, pyriform, amorphous, vacuolated (> 20% of area), reduced acrosome (< 40% of head area), absent acrosome (globozoospermia or round head syndrome), double head, pinhead
Neck and midpiece	absent tail, bent tail (> 90°), absent midpiece, irregular midpiece, abnormal thin midpiece
Tail	short, multiple, hairpin, broken (> 90°), irregular diameter, terminal droplet, coiled, Dag-defect
Immature forms	cytoplasmic droplets > 1/3 of spermhead area

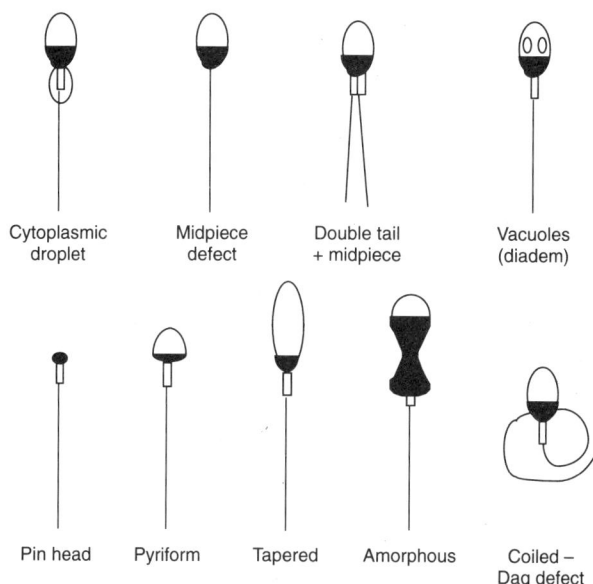

Figure 14 Some of the most common morphological abnormalities

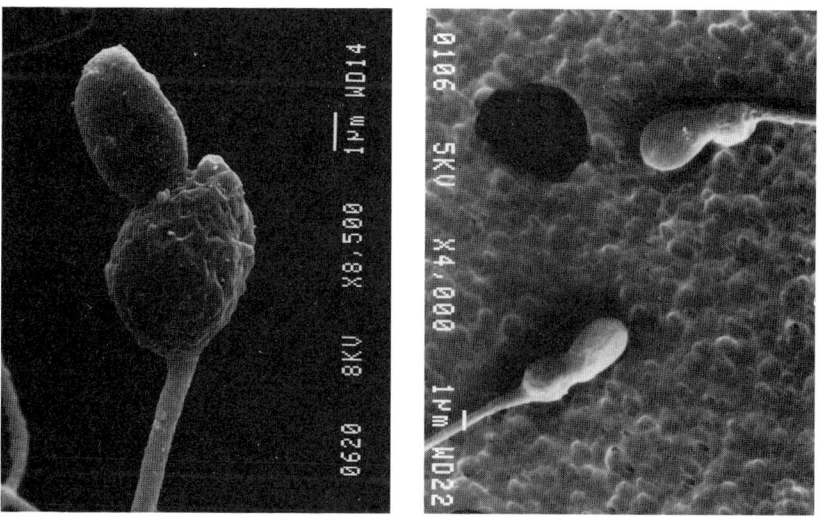

Figure 15 Scanning electron micrographs of the cytoplasmic droplet morphological abnormality

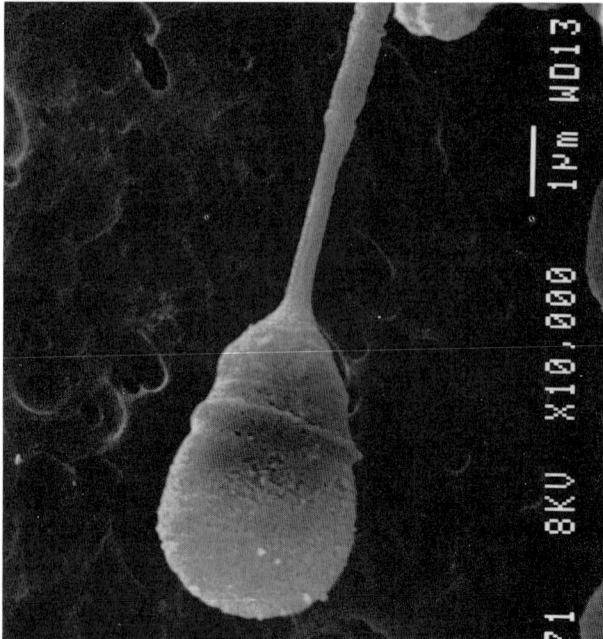

Figure 16 A scanning electron micrograph of the midpiece defect morphological abnormality

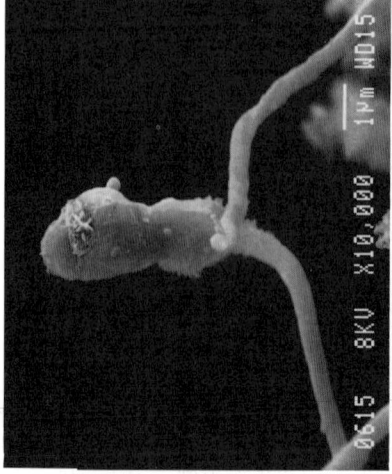
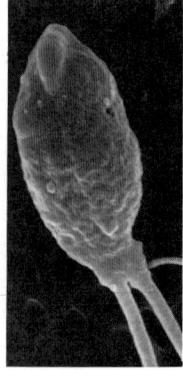

Figure 17 Scanning electron micrographs of two tail morphological abnormality. The sperm on the right also shows arrested cleavage

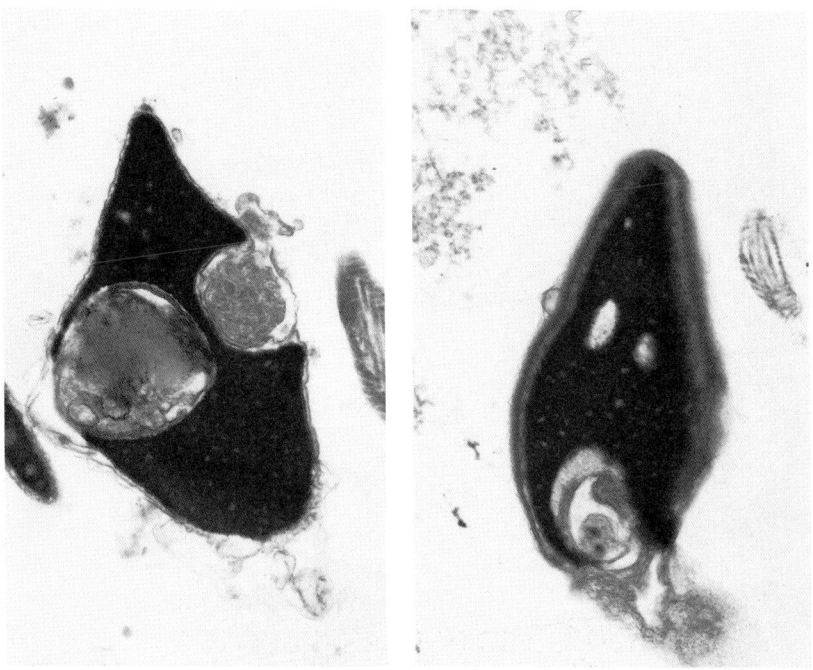

Figure 18   Transmission electron micrographs of diadem (vacuole) morphological abnormality

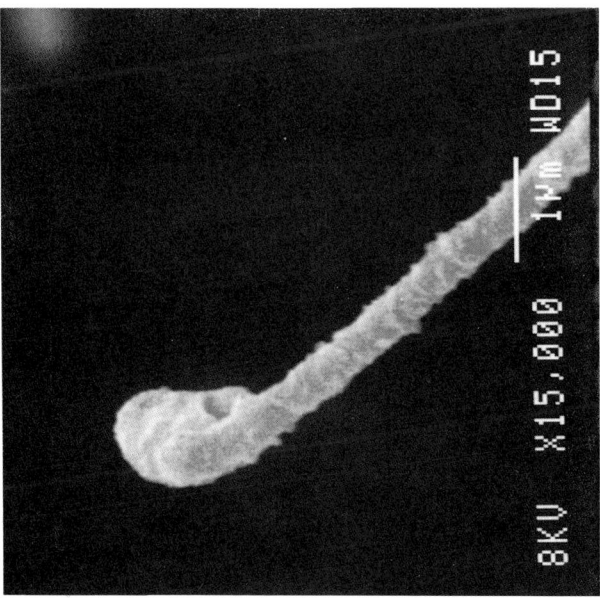

Figure 19   A scanning electron mmicrograph of 'pin head' morphological abnormality

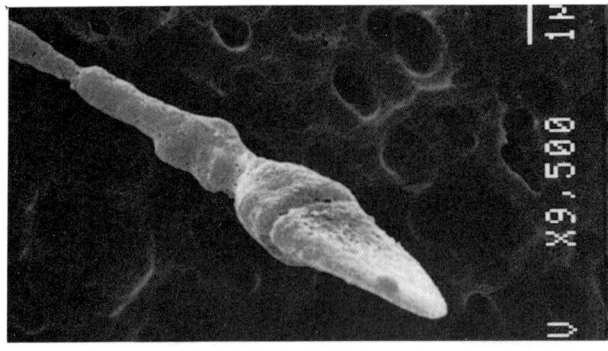

(A)

Figure 20 The tapered sperm head abnormality shown in a scanning electron micrograph (A) and tranmission electron micrograph (B)

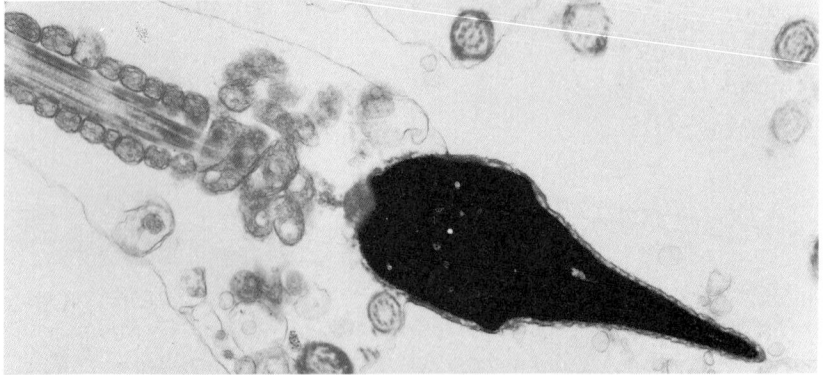

(B)

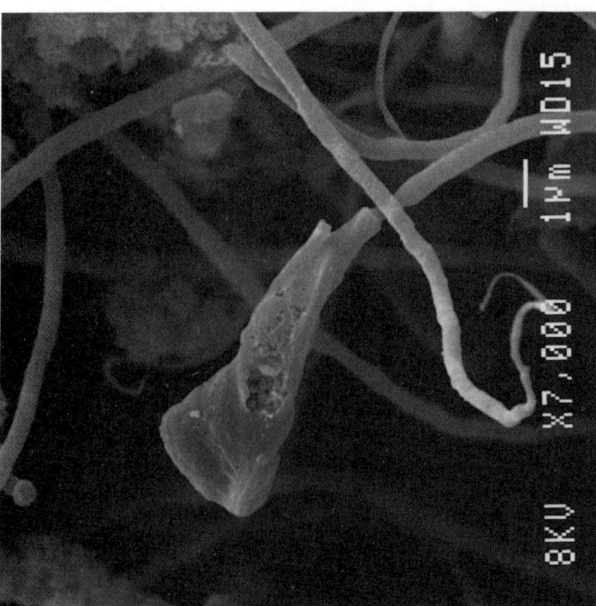

Figure 21 A scanning electron micrograph of amorphous morphological abnormality

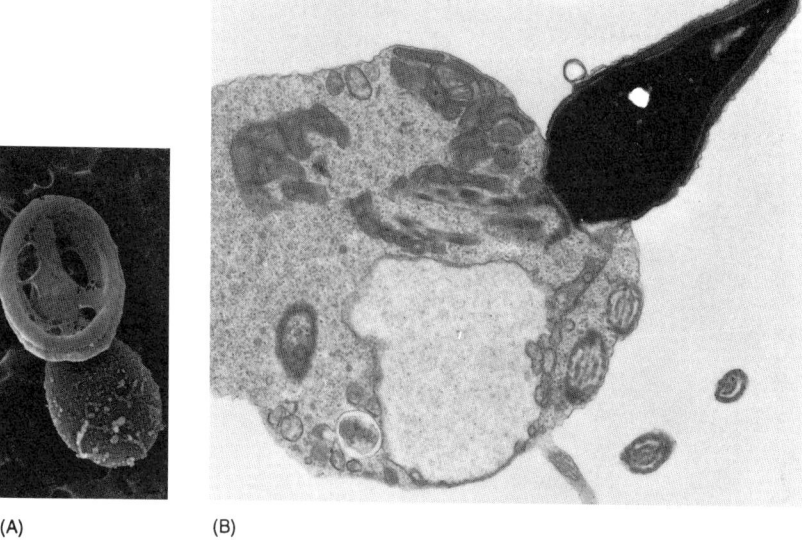

(A)   (B)

Figure 22   The Dag (coil) morphological abnormality shown on a scanning electron micrograph (A) and a transmission electron micrograph (B)

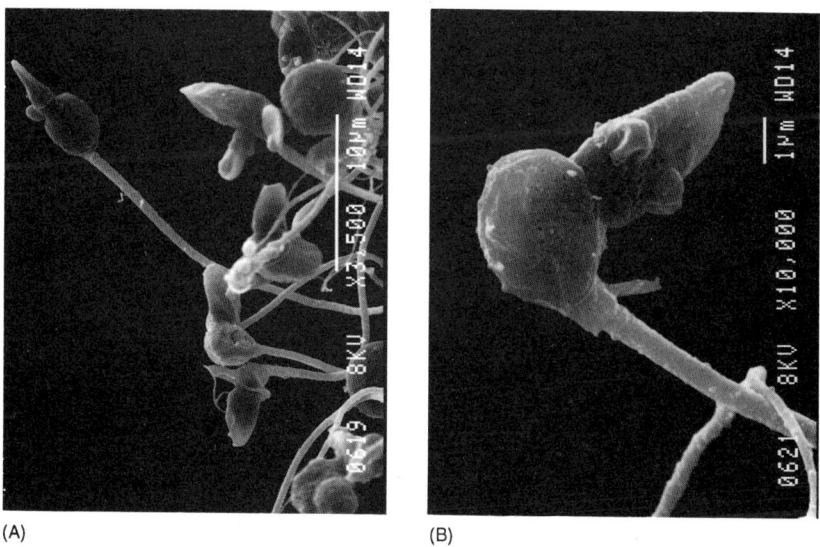

(A)   (B)

Figure 23   Sperm can show more than one morphological abnormality. These scanning electron micrographs show sperm with both tapered heads and cytoplasmic droplets. In addition the sperm in (B) is bent

1.   Jouannet, P., Ducot, B., Feneux, D. and Spira, A. (1988). Male factors and the likelihood of pregnancy in infertile couples. I. Study of sperm characteristics. *Int. J. Androl.*, **11**, 379

2. Kruger, T.F., DuToit. T.C., Franken, D.R., Acosta, A.A., Oehninger, S.C., Menkveld, R. and Lombard, C.J. (1993). A new computerized method of reading sperm morphology (strict criteria) is as efficient as technician reading. *Fertil. Steril.,.* 59, 202

3. Menkveld, R., Oettle, E.E., Krugerm T.F., Swanson, R.J., Acosta, A.A. and Oehninger, S. (1991). *Atlas of Human Sperm Morphology.* (Baltimore: Wiiliams and Wilkins)

4. World Health Organization (1992). *WHO Laboratory Manual For The Examination Of Human Semen And Sperm–Cervical Mucus Interaction,* 3rd edn. (Cambridge: Cambridge University Press)

Related subjects: morphology — normal, semen analysis — normal values, strict criteria, teratozoospermia

MORPHOLOGY, NORMAL

A normal human spermatozoon has an oval head, with a clear acrosomal and a darker postacrosomal region (see Figure 24). The tail (cross section shown Figure 25) is inserted in the head in a symmetrical way. The first part of the tail is slightly thickened and is called the midpiece. It should be realized that stained spermatozoa are slightly smaller than when viewed in wet preparations. Data of reported head size of normal spermatozoa are given in Table 24. Micrographs are shown in Figure 26.

According to the so-called strict criteria (Tygerberg, Kruger's) a normal spermatozoon should have the following characteristics:

(1) Smooth oval head 5–6 µm in length and 2.5–3.5 µm in diameter;

(2) Well defined acrosome involving 40–60% of the head;

(3) No defects of the midpiece or tail;

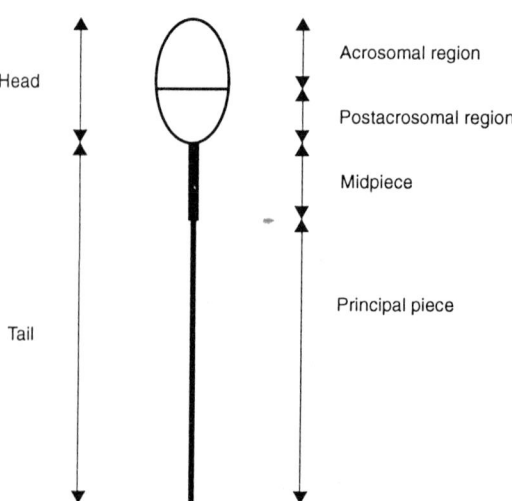

Figure 24   The different regions of a normal sperm

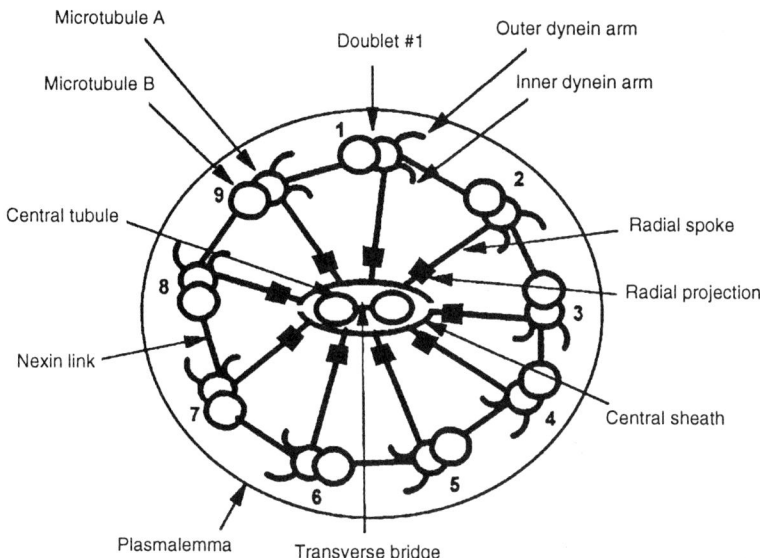

Figure 25 A transverse section of the axial filament showing the A9 + 2 axonemal complex. (Adapted from Mortimer, D.: *Practical Laboratory Andrology*. Oxford: Oxford University Press, 1994.)

Table 24 The normal measurements for spermatozoa

Parameter	Schrader	Strict criteria
Head length (μm)	4.57 ± 0.76	5.0–6.0
Head width (μm)	2.85 ± 0.42	2.5–3.5
Tail (whole length)	50 – 60 μm	

(4) No cytoplasmic droplets more than half the size of the sperm head; and

(5) Borderline forms are to be considered abnormal.

The shape, size and other characteristics of spermatozoa fertilizing the oocyte *in vivo* are not known. Therefore, the most frequent appearing morphological form in semen samples is taken as normal morphology. This concept is validated by the fact that spermatozoa drawn from mucus in the upper cervical canal generally have this typical appearance.

1. Kruger, T.F., Menkveld, R., Stander, F.S.H., Lombard, C.J., van der Merwe, J.P., van Zyl, J.A. and Smith, F. (1986). Sperm morphologic features as a prognostic factor in *in vitro* fertilization. *Fertil. Steril.*, 46, 1118

2. Oko, R. and Clermont, Y. (1990). Mammalian spermatozoa: structure and assembly of the tail. In Gagnon, C. (ed.) *Controls of Sperm Motility: Biological and Clinical Aspects.* (Boca Raton: CRC Press)

3. Schrader, S.M., Turner, T.W. and Simon, S.D. (1990). Longitudinal study of semen quality of unexposed workers: sperm head morphometry. *J. Androl.*, 11, 32

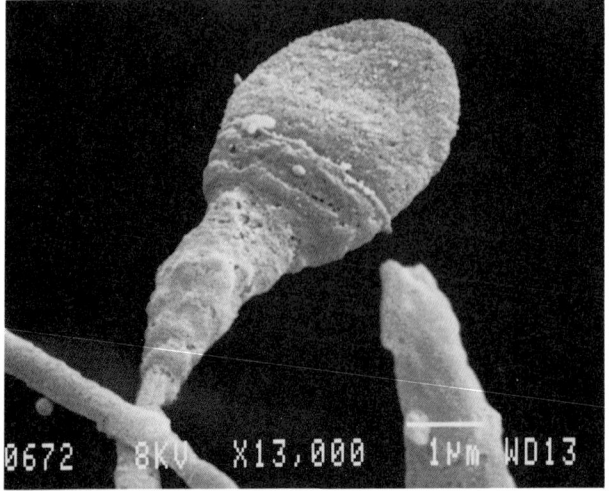

(A)

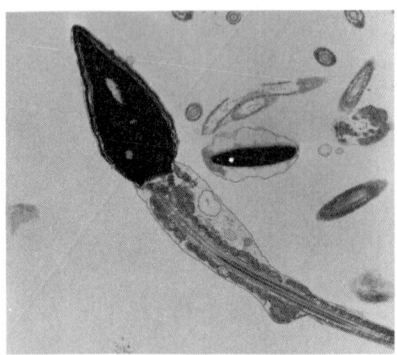

(B)

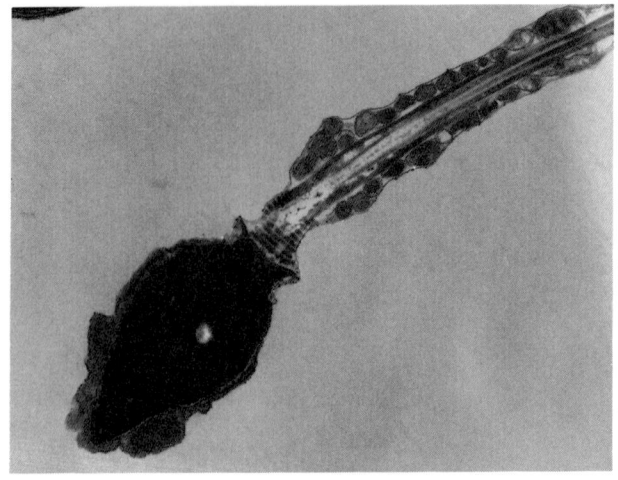

(C)

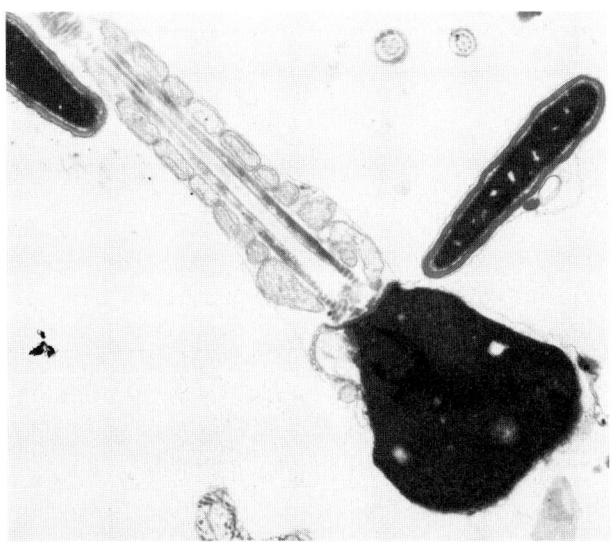

(D)

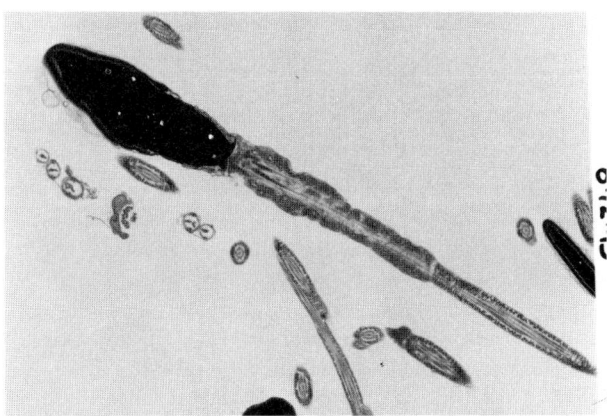

(E)

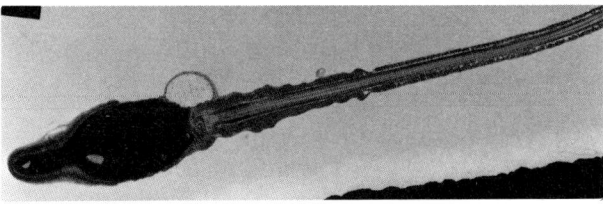

(F)

Figure 26 Normal sperm: (A) a scanning electron micrograph (SEM) of the head; (B) a transmission electron micrograph (TEM) of the head; (C) a TEM showing the connecting piece; (D and E) TEMs of the midpiece; and (F) a TEM of the tail

4. World Health Organization (1992). *WHO Laboratory Manual For The Examination Of Human Semen And Sperm–Cervical Mucus Interaction*, 3rd edn. (Cambridge: Cambridge University Press)

Related subjects: morphology — abnormal, semen analysis — normal values, strict criteria

MOTILITY

Spermatozoa have an intrinsic ability for motion usually referred to as motility. The spermatozoa acquire this motility by maturation during the passage through the epididymis. The energy needed for motility is produced in the mitochondria of the midpiece of the sperm. In the flagellum, adenosine triphosphate from the midpiece is hydroxylated into adenosine diphosphate (ADP) and monophosphate (AMP). The motility of a sperm sample can be described in terms of percentage of motile sperm in that sample (quantitative) or qualitative as a description of the type of motility exposed (e.g. progressive movements), speed (kinetics) or survival time of the motility *in vitro*. Since the motility of a spermatozoon is depending on the flagellar movement, nowadays it is technically possible to measure directly the flagellar movement patterns (e.g. beat frequency, wave length and wave amplitude). The major factors modulating axonemal motility appear to be cyclic AMP, calcium and protein phosphorylation. Spermatozoa themselves seem to release a factor into its environment (at least as shown in culture medium) which promotes motility. This motility enhancing factor had a maximum effect in media after 120 minutes of incubation.

1. Ishijima, S. and Mohri, H. (1990). Beating patterns of mammalian spermatozoa. In Gagnon, C. (ed.) *Controls of Sperm Motility: Biological and Clinical Aspects*. (Boca Raton: CRC Press)

2. Menkveld, R. and Kruger, T.F. (1990). Basic semen analysis. In Acosta, A.A. (ed.) *Human Spermatozoa in Assisted Reproduction*. (Baltimore: Williams and Wilkins)

3. Mortimer, D. (1994). Semen analysis. In Mortimer, D. (ed.) *Practical Laboratory Andrology*. (New York: Oxford University Press)

4. Shimonovitz, S., Ron, M., Manor, O., Har-Nir, R. and Hochner-Celnikier, D. (1995). Do spermatozoa secrete motility enhancing factor? *Fertil. Steril.*, 63(5), 1083

5. World Health Organization (1992). *WHO Laboratory Manual For The Examination Of Human Semen And Sperm–Cervical Mucus Interaction*, 3rd edn. (Cambridge: Cambridge University Press)

Related subjects: computer aided semen analysis, semen analysis — normal values, sperm maturation

MULLERIAN INHIBITING FACTOR (MIF)

This is the first (glyco)protein produced by the Sertoli cells after testicular differentiation has been initiated by the testis determining factor (TDF) located on the Y chromosome. It causes regression of the Mullerian ducts.

The Mullerian ducts are only sensitive to the factor during this brief period of time: after the end of the critical period, MIF no longer induces regression of the Mullerian ducts. MIF is possibly involved in the transabdominal part of the descent of the testicles from the posterior abdominal wall to the internal inguinal ring. In the literature MIF is sometimes referred to as anti-Mullerian hormone (AMH).

1. Josso, N. (1991). Anti-Mullerian hormone. In Robertson, D.M. and Herington, A.C. (eds.) Growth factors in endocrinology. *Bailliere's Clin. Endocrinol. Metab.*, 5(4), 635

Related subjects: embryology, testis determining factor, Y chromosome

MUMPS

Viral illness characterized by swelling of the salivary glands. Complications are rare in prepubertal boys. After puberty 10–35% of the cases are complicated by uni- or bilateral orchitis. The resulting testicular inflammation and edema within the firm and inelastic tunica albuginea results in pressure necrosis. The end stage is characterized by small testes, high levels of luteinizing hormone and follicle stimulating hormone and low testosterone. Testicular biopsy shows seminiferous tubular hyalinization and relative Leydig cell hyperplasia. Conservative management (bedrest, analgesics) results in 40–70% in testicular atrophy. Measures taken to reduce the incidence of atrophy include early incision of the tunica with drainage of the hydrocele and administration of 2B interferon. Proper vaccination programs for children can prevent mumps orchitis.

1. Erpenbach, K.H. (1991). Systemic treatment with interferon 2B: an effective method to prevent sterility after bilateral mumps orchitis. *J. Urol.*, 146, 54

2. Gerhard, I., Lenhard, K., Eggert-Kruse, W. and Runnebaum, B. (1992). Clinical data which influence semen parameters in infertile men. *Hum. Reprod.*, 7, 830

Related subjects: history — male infertility, hypergonadotropic hypogonadism, orchitis

MYCOPLASMA

Unique micro-organism with features characteristic of both bacteria and viruses. Some infected men have decreased semen parameters. The organism has also been incriminated in unexplained infertility. Doxycyclin is given as a treatment.

1. Moskowitz, M.O. and Mellinger, B.C. (1992). Sexually transmitted diseases and their relation to male infertility. *Urol. Clin. N. Am.*, 19(1), 35

Related subjects: sexually transmitted diseases

N*n*

NECROZOOSPERMIA

Only dead sperm cells are present in the semen sample. Sometimes necrozoospermia is difficult to distinguish from immotile but live spermatozoa. Supravital stains may not be very precise and reliable in distinguishing between the two. Only transmission electron microscopy is able to detect signs of cell death: fragmentation or disappearance of the plasma membrane, rarefaction of the acrosomal matrix, vesiculation of the peri-acrosomal membrane, extracellular dissolution of the acrosomal substance, karyolysis and swelling of the mitochondria.

1. Zamboni, L. (1992). Sperm structure and its relevance to infertility. An electron microscopic study. *Arch. Pathol. Lab. Med.*, 116(4), 325

Related subjects: asthenozoospermia, semen analysis — collection of sample, microscopy

NEEDLE BIOPSY, FINE NEEDLE ASPIRATION (FNA)

Percutaneous needle biopsy of the testes is an alternative to open testicular biopsy. At present, it is being introduced for standard clinical practice, since improvements in the design of the biopsy needles and devices have emerged. Comparisons between the histological diagnosis from tissue obtained with needle aspiration to open biopsy histology show good correlation in more than 90% of the specimen. In addition, the amount of tissue recovered is reported to be adequate. Fine needle biopsy thus seems to be an easy reproducible alternative to open biopsy, especially since it can be performed as an office procedure. It should be mentioned, however, that it is a blind procedure with possible unrecognized vascular and epididymal injuries.

1. Kessaris, D.N., Wasserman, P. and Mellinger, B.C. (1995). Histopathological and cytopathological correlations of percutaneous testis biopsy and open testis biopsy in infertile men. *J. Urol.*, 153(4), 1151

2. Mallidis, C. and Baker, H.W. (1994). Fine needle tissue aspiration biopsy of the testis. *Fertil. Steril.*, 61(2), 367

Related subjects: testicular biopsy, testicular biopsy — histopathology

NOONAN'S SYNDROME

Affected men present with short stature and webbed neck as in Turner's syndrome. Therefore the syndrome is somewhat misleadingly referred to as male Turner, since the karyotype is 46 XY. The majority of patients have cryptorchidism and diminished spermatogenesis, but fertility has been documented. Gonadotropin levels may be elevated, reflecting reduction in germ cell or Leydig cell function. Testicular biopsy reveals Sertoli cells only in the seminiferous tubules and reduced germ cells in other patients. The inheritance is likely to be autosomal dominant.

1. Sharland, M., Patton, M.A. and Burch, M. (1992). A clinical study of Noonan's syndrome. *Arch. Dis. Child.*, 67, 178

Related subjects: cryptorchidism, hypergonadotropic hypogonadism

NUTRITIONAL DEFICIENCIES

Sperm abnormalities in the form of maturation arrest at various levels are found in nutritional deficient conditions like alcohol abuse with liver cirrhosis, sickle-cell anemia and renal failure. Lack of vitamin A and zinc has been implemented in these conditions and normal vitamin and mineral status is therefore thought to be a prerequisite for normal spermatogenesis.

Related subjects: liver disease, renal failure, sickle-cell disease, zinc

NYCODENZ

A suspension of iohexol, a molecule used in radiology as an X-ray contrast medium (Omnipaque). It was introduced into the andrology laboratory because of concerns raised by the possible inflammatory reactions induced by Percoll-treated spermatozoa. Comparison of Percoll and Nycodenz gradients for sperm preparation shows comparable results.

1. Serafini, P., Blank, W., Tran, C., Mansourian, M., Tan, T. and Batzofin, J. (1990). Enhanced penetration of zona-free hamster ova by sperm prepared by Nycodenz and Percoll gradient centrifugation. *Fertil. Steril.*, 53, 551

Related subjects: Percoll, sperm preparation, swim-up

O_o

OBESITY

Obese infertile men differ from obese fertile and non-obese infertile men in their hormonal profile: they have low to normal luteinizing hormone and reduced serum sex hormone binding globulin and testosterone levels. These parameters and the testosterone/estradiol ratio seem to be the important markers of infertility. Increased aromatization of testosterone is one mechanism responsible, but weight loss does not restore estradiol levels to normal in spite of normal testosterone after weight loss.

1. Jarow, J.P., Kirkland, J., Koritnik, D.R. and Cefalu, W.T. (1993). Effect of obesity and fertility status on sex steroid levels in men. *Urology*, 42(2), 171

2. Strain, G.W., Zumoff, B., Miller, L.K., Rosner, W., Levit, C., Kalin, M., Hershcopf, R.J. and Rosenfeld, R.S. (1988). Effect of massive weightloss hypothalamic–pituitary–gonadal function in obese men. *J. Clin. Endocrinol. Metab.*, 66, 1019

Related subjects: endocrinology, testosterone, testosterone–estradiol binding globulin

OBSTRUCTION

Complete or partial obstruction of the sperm outflow tract can lead to azoospermia, oligozoospermia and a low (or sometimes normal) ejaculate volume with different findings for accessory gland markers. The categorization is shown in Table 25.

Related subjects: azoospermia, epididymis, congenital absence vas deferens, ejaculatory duct obstruction, oligozoospermia/low volume flowsheet, prostate, semen analysis — biochemical tests of seminal plasma, seminal vesicle, vasectomy reversal

OCCUPATIONAL HAZARDS

Exposure to heavy metals (e.g. cadmium, lead, mercury and manganese) may interfere with male reproductive function. The association between lead and impaired sperm parameters is relatively clear, for cadmium, mercury and manganese the association is much less obvious.

Exposure to electromagnetic fields has been associated with cancer, especially leukemia. No association has been reported between occupational

Table 25 The different types of obstruction to the sperm outflow tract

Place of obstruction	Cause	Epididymal markers	Seminal vesicle markers	Prostatic markers	Treatment
Epididymis	congenital	absent	present	present	artificial spermatocele; MESA, TESA
	infection	absent	present	present	Vasoepidymos-
	trauma	absent	present	present	tomy; artificial spermatocele; MESA, TESA
	post-vasectomy	absent	present	present	MESA, TESA
Vas deferens	vasectomy	absent	present	present	reversal of vasectomy; MESA, TESA
Ejaculatory duct	anatomic: infection, cysts	depending on site of and complete/ partial obstruction	depending on site of and complete/ partial obstruction	depending on site of and complete/ partial obstruction	transurethral surgery; MESA vibratory stimulation; electro-ejacu- lation; MESA
	functional: anejaculation				

MESA = microepididymal sperm aspirations, TESA = testicular sperm aspiration

exposure to high and medium magnetic fields and male reproductive function as reflected in semen parameters.

1. Gennart, J., Buchet, J. and Roels, H. (1992). Fertility of male workers exposed to cadmium, lead or manganese. *Am. J. Epidemiol.*, **135**, 208
2. Lundsberg, L.S., Bracken, M.B. and Belanger, K. (1995). Occupationally related magnetic field exposure and male subfertility. *Fertil. Steril.*, **63**(2), 384
3. McGregor, A.J. and Mason, M.J. (1990). Chronic occupational lead exposure and testicular endocrine function. *Hum. Exp. Toxicol.*, **9**, 371
4. Mohamed, M., Lee, W.I., Burbacher, T.M. and Mottet, N.K. (1986). Laser light-scattering sudy of the toxic effects of methylmercury on sperm motility. *J. Androl.*, **7**, 11

Related subjects: history — male infertility

OLIGOASTHENOTERATOZOOSPERMIA

Impaired spermatogenesis affects all semen properties, including count, motility and morphology. Therefore, oligoasthenozoospermia can be considered as a partial form of spermatogenic arrest.

Related subjects: history — male infertility, oligoasthenoteratozoospermia — flowsheet, physical examination — male infertility, semen analysis — normal values, spermatogenic arrest

OLIGOASTHENOZOOSPERMIA, FLOWSHEET DIAGNOSIS AND MANAGEMENT (Figure 27)

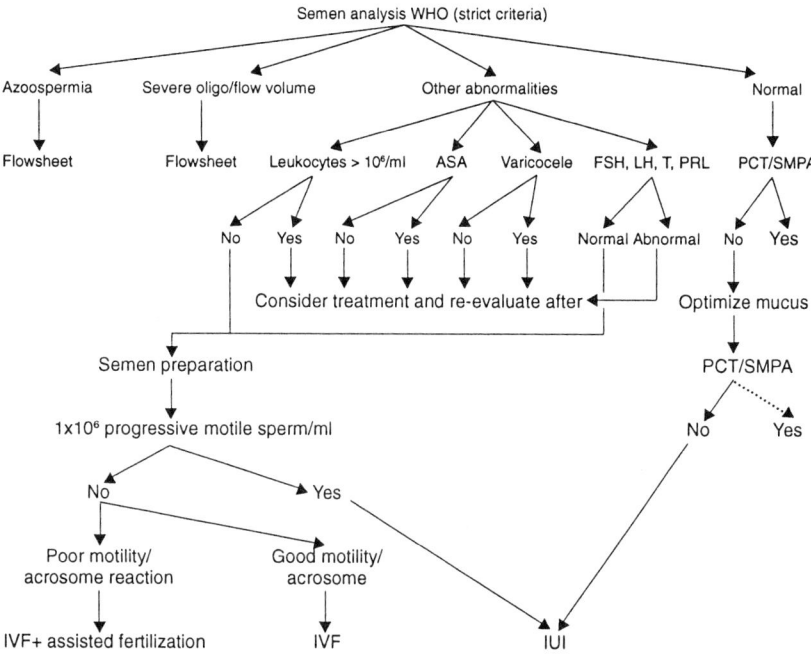

Figure 27 As a guideline for male infertility work-up with the semen analysis as a starting point, the following algorithm can be utilized. It is important to stress the necessity to include a detailed history and perform a physical examination. WHO = World Health Organization, ASA = antisperm antibodies, FSH = follicle stimulating hormone, LH = luteinizing hormone, PRL = prolactin, T = testosterone, PCT = postcoital test, SMPA = sperm mucus penetration assay, IVF = *in vitro* fertilization, IUI = intrauterine insemination

Related subjects: acrosome reaction test, antisperm antibodies test, azoospermia — flowsheet, hypogonadotropic hypogonadism, leukocytospermia, oligozoospermia/low volume flowsheet, postcoital test, varicocele

OLIGOZOOSPERMIA

All semen parameters are normal, except the number of spermatozoa. The total ejaculate is below 40 million or less than 20 million per ml (World Health Organization). Oligospermia may be caused by malformation or partial obstruction of the ejaculatory ducts. Often oligozoospermia is present in combination with asthenozoospermia.

1. Menkveld, R. and Kruger, T.F. (1990). Basic semen analysis. In Acosta, A.A. (ed.) *Human Spermatozoa In Assisted Reproduction.* (Baltimore: Williams and Wilkins)

2. Mortimer, D. (1994). Semen analysis. In Mortimer, D. (ed.) *Practical Laboratory Andrology.* (New York: Oxford University Press)

3. World Health Organization (1992). *WHO Laboratory Manual for the Examination of Human Semen and Sperm–Cervical Mucus Interaction,* 3rd edn. (Cambridge: Cambridge University Press)

Related subjects: history — male infertility, physical examination — male infertility, oligozoospermia/low volume — flowsheet, semen analysis — normal values

OLIGOZOOSPERMIA/LOW VOLUME, FLOWSHEET DIAGNOSIS AND MANAGEMENT (Figure 28)

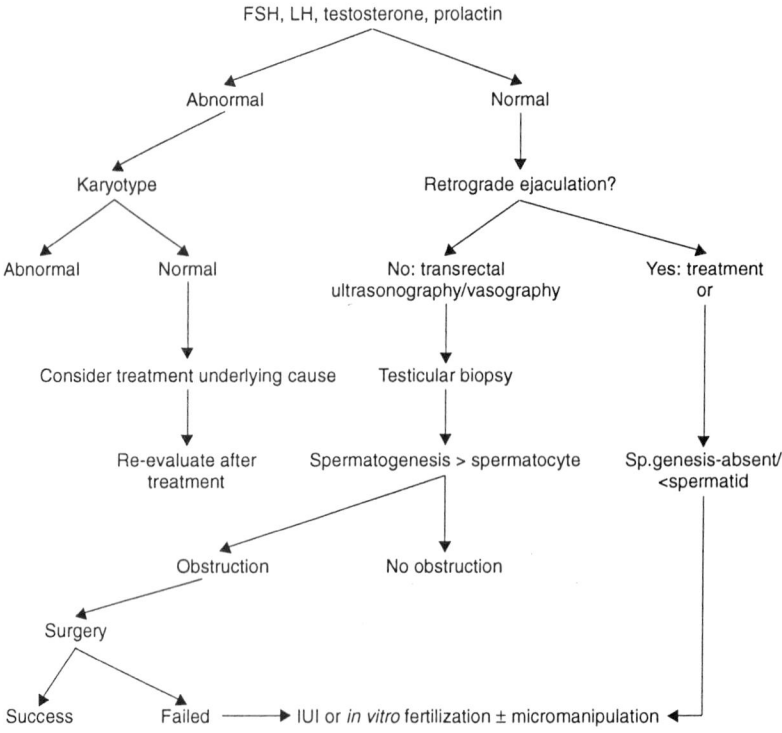

Figure 28   Severe oligozoospermia can be defined as number of spermatozoa < 5 million/ml. A volume below 1.5 ml is supposed to be abnormal. This flow chart provides guidelines on its diagnosis and management. FSH = follicle stimulating hormone, LH = luteinizing hormone, IUI = intrauterine insemination

Related subjects: hypogonadotropic hypogonadism, obstruction, spermatogenesis — testicular biopsy

OOLEMMA

The egg-plasma membrane: it is the primary location of fusion of the acrosome reacted sperm and the oocyte.

Related subjects: fertilization

ORCHIDOPEXY

Surgical correction of undescended testicle(s). The fertility prognosis is poor with bilateral undescended testes, but somewhat better if the condition is unilateral and if orchidopexy is performed between 1 and 2 years of age. In addition, the original anatomical position of the testes – abdominal, cannalicular or inguinal – is of prognostic importance. The final testicular volume correlates well with sperm variables. Patients with a history of cryptorchidism usually have a high percentage of antisperm antibodies (60%), contributing to reduced fertility.

1. Cendron, M., Keating, M.A. and Huff, D.S. (1989). Cryptorchidism, orchiopexy and infertility: a critical longterm retrospective analysis. Part II. *J. Urol.*, 142, 559

2. Mandat, K.M., Wieczorkiewicz, B., Gubala-Kacala, M., Sypniewski, J. and Bujok, G. (1994). Semen analysis of patients who had orchidopexy in childhood. *Eur. J. Pediatr. Surg.*, 4(2), 94

3. Urry, R.L., Carrell, D.T., Starr, N.T., Snow, B.W. and Middleton, R.G. (1994). The incidence of antisperm antibodies in infertility patients with a history of cryptorchidism. *J. Urol.*, 151(2), 381

Related subjects: antisperm antibodies, cryptorchidism, retractile testis, scrotal temperature

ORCHITIS

Inflammation of the testicles causing temporary or long-term defective spermatogenesis. May be caused by infections (bacterial, viral, e.g. mumps), autoimmune disorder or radiation.

Related subjects: history — male infertility, hypergonadotropic hypogonadism, mumps, radiation

OXYGEN, REACTIVE SPECIES

The presence of reactive oxygen species, liberated by activated leukocytes or by immature spermatozoa cause peroxidation of the polyunsaturated fatty acids of the sperm plasma membrane, which may result in loss of membrane fluidity. Spermatozoa are very susceptible to such damage because of the fact that they contain many unsaturated fatty acids. This vulnerability is increased by the fact that spermatozoa have limited amounts of protective enzymes such as superoxide dismutase and glutathione peroxidase. Abnormal exposition to reactive oxygen species may therefore result in loss of normal sperm motility and failure to undergo the normal acrosome reaction, which is a prerequisite to oocyte fusion.

1. Aitken, J. and Fisher, H. (1994). Reactive oxygen species generation and human spermatozoa: the balance of benefit and risk. *Bioessays*, 16(4), 259

Related subjects: acrosome reaction, antioxidants, leukocytospermia, sperm preparation

P*p*

PARAPLEGIA

There is impaired ability to have intravaginal ejaculation and sperm motility is decreased. Testicular biopsies show atrophy. This is partly secondary to destruction of sympathetic innervation.

1. Chapelle, P.A., Roby-Brami, A., Jondet, M., Piechaud, T. and Bussel, B. (1993). Trophic effects on testes in paraplegics. *Paraplegia*, 31(9), 576

Related subjects: electro-ejaculation, retrograde ejaculation, spinal cord injury, vibratory stimulation

PARTIAL ZONA DISSECTION (PZD)

Part of the oocyte zona pellucida is cut with a glass needle or a metal microblade in order to circumvent one selection barrier for the spermatozoon in the process of fertilization. Another selection barrier, the vitelline membrane, is present. Abnormal hatching has been observed after the procedure.

1. Cohen, J., Malter, H., Wright, G., Elsner, C., Kort, K. and Massey, J. (1988). Implantation of embryos after partial opening of oocyte zona pellucida to facilitate sperm penetration. *Lancet*, ii, 162

2. Vanderzwalmen, P., Barlow, P., Nijs, M., Bertin, G., Leroy, F. and Schoysman, R. (1992). Usefulness of partial zona dissection in a human *in vitro* fertilization programme. *Hum. Reprod.*, 7, 537

Related subjects: intracytoplasmic sperm injection, micromanipulation, subzonal insemination, zona drilling

PENTOXIFYLLINE

Methyl xanthine derivate in the same pharmacological class as caffeine and theophylline. It is thought to reduce blood viscosity, to increase erythrocyte flexibility and improve testicular microcirculation. It is also a phosphodiesterase inhibitor, resulting in increased intracellular cyclic adenosine monophosphate. This in turn increases cellular glycolysis and endogenous adenosine triphosphate production, which is thought to increase sperm motility. Oral administration of pentoxifylline to patients with idiopathic oligospermia shows conflicting results. It might be effective *in vitro* where it has improved fertilization in a subset of patients with insufficient acrosomal reaction. There is some concern that it could be embryotoxic.

1. Carver-Ward, J.A., Jaroudi, K.A., Einspenner, M., Parhar, R.S., Al-Sedairy, S.T. and Sheth, K.V. (1994). Pentoxifylline potentiates ionophore (A23187) mediated acrosome reaction in human sperm: flow cytometric analysis using CD46 antibody. *Hum. Reprod.*, 9(1), 71

2. Tesarik, J. and Mendoza, C. (1993). Sperm treatment with pentoxifylline improves the fertilizing ability in patients with acrosome reaction insufficiency. *Fertil. Steril.*, 60, 141

3. Tournaye, H., van Steirteghem, A.C. and Devroey, P. (1994). Pentoxifylline in idiopathic male-factor infertility: a review of its therapeutic efficacy after oral administration. *Hum. Reprod.*, 9(6), 996

4. Wang, C., Chan, C. and Wong, K. (1983). Comparison of the effectiveness of placebo, clomiphene citrate, mesterolone, pentoxifylline and testosterone rebound therapy for the treatment of idiopathic oligospermia. *Fertil. Steril.*, 40, 358

5. Yovich, J.L. (1993). Pentoxifylline: actions and applications in assisted reproduction. *Hum. Reprod.*, 8(11), 1786

Related subjects: medication — treatment

PERCOLL

A suspension of colloidal silica particles conjugated to povidone. Continuous or discontinuous Percoll gradients are used for sperm separation on the basis of differences in cell density. Normal sperm heads and midpieces have a higher density than those with head and midpiece anomalies. Therefore, spermatozoa with normal head and neck morphology are present to a higher degree in the concentrated fractions of the Percoll gradient. Sperm preparation with Percoll has been reported to yield better recovery of viable motile spermatozoa than with wash and swim-up methods. Spermatozoa prepared by Percoll are largely free of bacteria and leukocytes. Theoretical concerns about the use of Percoll have been the presence of small quantities of the material in the prepared spermatozoa, as well as the occasional finding of endotoxins.

1. Hall, J.A., Fishel, S.B., Timson, J.A., Dowell, K. and Klentzeris, L.D. (1995). Human sperm morphology evaluation pre- and post-Percoll gradient centrifugation. *Hum. Reprod.*, 10

2. Jaroudi, K.A., Carver-Ward, J.A., Hamilton, C.J.C.M., Sieck, U.V. and Sheth, K.V. (1993). Percoll semen preparation enhances human oocyte fertilization in male factor infertility as shown by a randomized cross-over study. *Hum. Reprod.*, 8, 1438

3. Menkveld, R., Swanson, R.J., Kotze, V.W. and Kruger, T.F. (1990). Comparison of a discontinuous Percoll gradient method versus a swim-up method: effects on sperm morphology and other semen parameters. *Andrologia*, 22, 152

4. Mortimer, D. (1990). Semen analysis and sperm washing techniques. In Gagnon, C. (ed.) *Controls of Sperm Motility: Biological and Clinical Aspects.* (Boca Raton: CRC Press)

Related subjects: Nycodenz, sperm preparation, swim-up

PERCUTANEOUS EPIDIDYMAL SPERM ASPIRATION (PESA)

The method by which epididymal spermatozoa are collected using a small needle to which suction is connected. This technique is blind in contrast to the microsurgical approach of the epididymis. First reports mention good results, especially when the sperm thus obtained were used in combination with *in vitro* fertilization and intracytoplasmic sperm injection. If the procedure proves to be of value, repetitive scrotal and epididymal surgery can be avoided.

1. Craft, I., Tsirigotis, M., Bennett, V., Taranissi, M., Khalifa, Y., Hogewind, G. and Nicholson, N. (1995). Percutaneous epididymal sperm aspiration and intracytoplasmic sperm injection in the management of infertilty due to obstructive azoospermia. *Fertil. Steril.*, 63(5), 1038

Related subjects: azoospermia, micro-epididymal sperm aspiration, testicular sperm aspiration

PESTICIDES

For many pesticides animal data concerning reproductive toxicity are not available and, for most, human data are lacking. A major problem in the evaluation of of toxic substances and their effect on reproduction is multiple exposure. Contamination with many different compounds at the same time is common. An important feature of possibly harmful substances is their half-life. Organochlorine components, for example, to which many insecticides, fungicides and herbicides belong, have an extremely long retention time in body tissues. Some of the substances and their effect on semen are listed in Table 26.

Table 26   The effect of pesticides on semen

Type	Effect
Dibromochloropropane	oligospermia, azoospermia, decreased motility, higher than expected female births, increase in abortions in female partners
Chlordecone	oligospermia, decreased motility
Ethylene dibromide	decreased count and motility, increased abnormal morphology
Carbaryl	increased abnormal morphology
2,4 D	decreased count and motility, increased abnormal morphology

1. Feichtinger, W. (1991). Environmental factors and fertility. *Hum. Reprod.*, 6(8), 1170

2. Mattison, D.R., Bogumil, R.J. and Chapin, R. (1990). Reproductive effects of pesticides.

In: Baker, S.R. and Wilkinson, C.F. (eds.) *The Effects of Pesticides on Human Health. Advances in Modern Environmental Toxicology.* (Princeton CJ, Princeton Scientific)

3. Weisenburger, D.D. (1993). Human health effects of agrichemical use. *Hum. Pathol.*, 24, 571

Related subjects: history — male infertility, hypergonadotropic hypogonadism

PHYSICAL ENDURANCE

Endurance athletes have low levels of both total and free testosterone and alterations in luteinizing hormone release. For endurance runners, conflicting results have been reported regarding sperm density, morphology and motility, but in general endurance sport does not seem to affect fertility.

1. Arce, J.C., De Souza, M.J., Pescatello, L.S. and Luciano, A.A. (1993). Subclinical alterations in hormone and semen profile in athletes. *Fertil. Steril.*, 59, 398

2. Bagatell, C.J. and Bremner, W.J. (1990). Sperm counts and reproductive hormones in male marathoners and lean controls. *Fertil. Steril.*, 53(4), 688

Related subjects: endocrinology

PHYSICAL EXAMINATION, IN MALE INFERTILITY (Table 27)

A complete physical examination should be part of the work-up of male infertility as it may direct attention towards the underlying pathology and/ or systemic disease.

Related subjects: history — male infertility

POOR PROGNOSIS PATTERN OF MORPHOLOGY

Patients who are showing less than 4% normal forms according to Kruger's strict criteria have a poor prognosis. In regular *in vitro* fertilization, this group has a fertilization rate of less than 10%.

1. Kruger, T.F., Acosta, A.A., Simmons, K.F., Swanson, J.R., Matta, J.F. and Oehninger, S. (1988). Predictive value of abnormal sperm morphology in *in vitro* fertilization. *Fertil. Steril.*, 49, 112

Related subjects: morphology — normal, morphology — abnormal, strict criteria

POSTCOITAL TEST

Evaluation of sperm ability to penetrate into pre-ovulatory mucus 2–12 h after intercourse. Mucus collected from the endocervix is evaluated and the number of progressive motile sperm in 10 randomly chosen high-power fields (400×) are counted. Opinion about the value of the test is divided. Review of the literature shows sensitivity ranging from 0.09 to

Table 27 The factors checked in a complete physical examination of a man who presents with male infertility

General	habitus	possible chromosomal or hormonal abnormalities
	body mass index	obesity can cause hormonal disturbances
	blood pressure	high blood pressure can be caused by renal disease
Secondary sex characteristics	hair growth	hormonal abnormalities
	muscle development	hormonal abnormalities
	breasts	hyperprolactinemia
Penis	length	hypogonadism
	hypo/epispadia	associated congenital abnormalities
	phimosis	
	circumcision	
Scrotum	thickness of skin	
Testis	volume	hypogonadotrophy/atrophy of germ cells and seminiferous tubules
	consistency	decrease in mumps atrophy; increase in Klinefelter atrophy
	position	maldescent; cryptorchidism; retractile
Epididymis	size	cyst
	consistency	increase after infections
Vas deferens	present (±)	congenital absence
	irregularities	postinfection
Varicocele	present (±)	grading of varicocele
	Valsalva maneuver (±)	
Hydrocele	present (±)	
	size	
Prostate	size	enlarged
	tender	infection
Seminal vesicle	palpable (±)	normally not palpable

0.71, specificity from 0.62 to 1.00, positive predictive value from 0.25 to 0.75 and negative predictive value from 0.56 to 1.00. Apart from this, there is no consensus regarding standard methodology and uniform definition of normality. Within a setting using strict protocols, however, the test is a good predictor of pregnancy within the first year after intake for infertility evaluation.

1. Eimers, J.M., te Velde, J.R., Gerritse, R., van Kooy, R.J., Kremer, J. and Habbema, J.D. (1994). The validity of the postcoital test for estimating the probability of conceiving. *Am. J. Obstet. Gynecol.*, 171(1), 65

2. Griffith, C.S. and Grimes, D.A. (1990). The validity of the postcoital test. *Am. J. Obstet. Gynecol.*, 162(3), 615

3. Hull, M.G.R., Savage, P.E. and Bromham, D.R. (1982). Prognostic value of the postcoital test: prospective study based on time-specific conception rates. *Br. J. Obstet. Gynaecol.*, 89, 299

Related subjects: sperm function test, Kremer test, Kurzrok–Miller test, Sims–Huhner test, sperm–cervical mucus contact test

PRO-ACROSIN

The inactive form of acrosin, which becomes partly activated during the acrosome reaction.

Related subjects: acrosin, acrosome reaction

PROLACTIN

Prolactin is a polypeptide hormone that is produced in the lateral part of the anterior pituitary. Plasma levels in males are the same or slightly lower than in females. It potentiates the effect of luteinizing hormone on the Leydig cells and specifically the testosterone secretion. Testosterone and prolactin synergize in the stimulation of other tissues in the male genital tract. Testosterone and estradiol stimulate prolactin secretion. Possibly there is a direct effect of prolactin on the brain influencing behavior, as has been suggested in hyperprolactinemic men.

1. Catt, K.J. and Dufau, M.L. (1991). Gonadotropic hormones: biosynthesis, secretion, receptors and actions. In Yen, S.S.C. and Jaffe, R.B. (eds.) *Reproductive Endocrinology*, 3rd edn. (Philadelphia: W.B. Saunders)

Related subjects: endocrinology, hyperprolactinemia, microadenoma

PROSTAGLANDINS

The prostaglandins in seminal fluid are almost exclusively derived from the seminal vesicles. Primarily prostaglandin E_2 and 19 OH E_2 are concerned. A suggested function of prostaglandins is stimulation of sperm motility.

1. Cooper, T.G., Yeung, C.H., Nashan, D. and Nieschlag, E. (1988). Epididymal markers in human infertility. *J. Androl.*, 9, 91

Related subjects: semen analysis — biochemical test of seminal plasma, seminal vesicle

PROSTATE

The prostate is 3.5–4.0 cm in diameter and located around the urethra below the bladder neck. It has a multiglandular function. It has, for example, exclusive secretion of acid phosphatase, zinc, citric acid and fibrinolytic enzymes responsible for the liquefaction of coagulated vesicular secretion. It provides the first fraction of the ejaculate and constitutes 30% of its volume. In addition, it carries the major fraction of spermatozoa from an ejaculate.

1. Mortimer, D. (1994). *Practical Laboratory Andrology*. (Oxford: Oxford University Press)

Related subjects: anatomy, ejaculate — composition, liquefaction, semen analysis — biochemical test of seminal plasma

PROSTATITIS, BACTERIAL

Acute bacterial prostatitis is usually a self-limiting disease which is effectively treated with parenteral broad spectrum antibiotics. Chronic bacterial prostatitis is difficult to treat, as the causative micro-organism(s) often persist in the prostatic tissue and fluid and thus may lead to relapsing urogenital tract infections with negative repercussions for semen quality due to leukocytospermia. Sometimes prostatitis can be diagnosed by the Stamey–Meares test. In this test three fractionated urine samples are analyzed: the first one is indicative for the urethra, the second can be considered as a midstream urine and so is representative for urinary tract infection. Finally, the third one is obtained after prostatic massage and indicates prostatic infection. The test is positive if the third sample contains at least ten times more bacteria as the first fraction. Co-trimoxazole, and recently more successfully the newer quinolones such as norfloxacin and ciprofloxacin, are used for treatment.

1. ESHRE Capri Workshop Group (1994). Male sterility and subfertility: guidelines for management. *Hum. Reprod.*, 9(7), 1260
2. Naber, K.G. (1991). The role of quinolones in the treatment of chronic bacterial prostatitis. *Infection*, 19 (Suppl. 3), S170

Related subjects: bacterial infection, culture semen, leukocytospermia, medication — treatment

PROSTATITIS, NON-BACTERIAL

Chronic non-bacterial prostatitis is a relative common disorder associated with higher prevalence of antisperm antibodies and an excessive production of reactive oxygen species. Sperm motility and normal morphology are found to be decreased. There is a strong correlation between the duration of the disease and the morphological defects.

1. Christiansen, E., Tollefsrud, A. and Purvis, K. (1991). Sperm quality in men with chronic abacterial prostatovesiculitis verified by rectal ultrasonography. *Urology*, 38(6), 545
2. Leib, Z., Bartoov, B., Eltes, F. and Servadio, C. (1994). Reduced semen quality caused by chronic abacterial prostatitis: an enigma or reality? *Fertil. Steril.*, 61(6), 1109–16

Related subjects: antisperm antibodies, bacterial infection, culture semen, leukocytospermia

PROTEIN CARBOXYL METHYLASE (PCM) ENZYME

Protein carboxyl methylase is an enzyme that methylates free carboxyl groups of proteins. It is involved in different forms of cell motility. In the spermatozoon the highest concentration is found in the sperm tail. PCM deficiency is restricted to spermatozoa only, suggesting a post-translational genetic defect. The literature is controversial about the significance of measurement of protein carboxyl methylase in infertility patients.

1. Gagnon, C., de Lamirande, E. and Sherins, R.J. (1986). Positive correlation between the level of protein-carboxyl methylase in spermatozoa and sperm motility. *Fertil. Steril.*, 45, 847

Related subjects: asthenozoospermia, motility

Qq

QUINOLONE DERIVATES

Group of antibiotics (e.g. pefloxacine, ofloxacin, fleroxacin and ciprofloxacin) developed for treatment of urogenital infections. Indicated specifically in treatment of acute and chronic male accessory gland infection because of their high concentrations in semen, prostate and seminal vesicles. They are also very effective in treatment of chlamydial urethritis.

1. Fitton, A. (1992). The quinolones. An overview of their pharmacology. *Clin. Pharmacokinet.*, **22** (Suppl. 1), 11

2. Naber, K.G. (1991). The role of quinolones in the treatment of chronic bacterial prostatitis. *Infection*, **19** (Suppl. 3), S170-7

Related subjects: antibiotics — effect on spermatogenesis, culture semen, medication — treatment, prostatitis

R *r*

RADIATION EXPOSURE

Radiation exposure, as employed in radiotherapy, has spermatotoxic effects varying with the dose and the duration of treatment. Radiation has its greatest effects on the less differentiated cells: type B spermatogonia are the most radiosensitive, spermatocytes are 10 times and spermatids even 40 times more resistant. In addition, spermatozoa and Leydig cells are relatively protected. Until these mature forms are depleted, fecundity is often maintained. Protection of spermatogenesis against cytotoxicity by androgen deprivation through suppression with luteinizing hormone releasing hormone analogue or combinations of androgens and progestogens has not been observed in the human. If post-meiotic cells survive, there is a great risk of induced chromosomal abnormalities. After this period, there is often a temporary or permanent azoospermia. Due to the relative resistance of Leydig cells to radiation, sometimes a monotropic rise in follicle stimulating hormone is observed. Recovery will occur depending on the dose delivered to the testis:

(1) < 100 cGY: 9–18 months;

(2) 200–300 cGY: to 30 months;

(3) 400–600 cGY: > 5 years; and

(4) > 600 cGy: permanent sterility.

Some concern is justified about environmental pollution with radionuclides. Some of these long-lived substances can be deposited in human tissues. The radioactive isotopes caesium-134 and caesium-137 were present in the majority of the seminal fluid samples, investigated after the Chernobyl reactor accident.

1. Feichtinger, W. (1991). Environmental factors and fertility. *Hum. Reprod.*, 6(8), 1170

2. Hahn, E.W., Feingold, S.M. and Simpson, L. (1987). Recovery from aspermia induced by low dose radiation in seminoma patients. *Cancer*, 47, 2368

3. Krenn, C.G., Herczeg, K., Albrecht, A., Koppensteiner, E., Mikoleit, B., Rahmani, A., Stranzinger, J., Weichselberger, A., Wieser, S., Unfried, E. and Feichtinger, W. (1990). Radioaktives Caesium 137 und Caesium 134 in der Follikel- und Samenflussigkeit. *Geburtdhilfe Frauenheilkd.*, 50, 394

4. Morris, I.D. (1993). Protection agianst cytotoxic induced testis damage – experimental approaches. *Eur. Urol.*, 23(1), 143

5.   Rowley, M.J., Leach, D.R. and Warner, G.A. (1974). Effects of graded doses of ionizing radiation on the human testis. *Radiat. Res.*, 59, 665

Related subjects: azoospermia, chromosomal abnormalities — sperm cells, germ cell mutagens, hypergonadotropic hypogonadism, spermatogenesis, spermatogenic arrest, testicular cancer

REDUCTASE DEFICIENCY, 5α

The syndrome is characterized by a deficiency in the 5α-reductase enzyme which converts testosterone intracellularly into dihydrotestosterone. The result is male pseudohermaphroditism with some resemblance to androgen insensitivity syndrome. The disease, however, is autosomal recessive and the abnormality is not present in the androgen receptor. Structures dependent on testosterone presence are developed – Wolffian ducts derivatives seminal vesicles, ejaculatory ducts, epididymis and vas deferens – whereas dihydrotestosterone dependent structures, including external genitalia, urethra and prostate, are not developed in the male. Further characteristics at birth include hypospadia, female external genitalia and failure of labioscrotal fusion. At puberty masculinization occurs, breasts remain male and there is decreased to normal testicular function.

1.   Speroff, L., Glass, R.H. and Kase, N.G. (1994). *Clinical Gynecologic Endocrinology and Infertility*, 5th edn. (Baltimore: Williams and Wilkins)

Related subjects: androgen insensitivity, embryology, testicular feminization

RENAL FAILURE

There is lack of progression in spermatogenesis beyond the primary spermatocyte stage. One of the possible etiological factors is thought to be zinc deficiency. Testosterone levels are decreased and follicle stimulating hormone and luteinizing hormone elevated. The elevated level of luteinizing hormone is due to a decreased metabolic clearance rate.

Since the major defect involves hypothalamic dysfuction, however, the result is a relative hypogonadotropism. Following dialysis testosterone increases, but usually not to the normal range.

1.   Mahajan, S.K., Abasi, A.A., Prasad, A.S., Rabani, P., Briggs, W.A. and McDonald, F.D. (1982). Effects of oral zinc therapy on gonadal function in hemodialysis patients. *Ann. Int. Med.*, 97, 357

2.   Martin-du-Pan, R.C. and Campana, A. (1993). Physiopathology of spermatogenic arrest. *Fertil. Steril.*, 60(6), 937

Related subjects: hypergonadotropic hypogonadism, nutritional deficiencies, spermatogenic arrest, zinc

RETRACTILE TESTIS

Retractile testis are easily withdrawn from the intrascrotal position to a higher location due to the cremasteric reflex. This reflex is supposed to disappear 1–2 years before puberty. In a male infertility population up to 4% of men are reported to have retractile testis. In these patients abnormal histology on testicular biopsy has been found. Semen parameters include abnormal count, motility and morphology. Follicle stimulating hormone levels are normal or elevated. Scrotal orchidopexy has to be considered in case of abnormal semen parameters and infertility, although no prospective studies have been performed.

1. Jarrett, T.W., Mininberg, D.T. and Goldstein, M. (1992). Infertility in patients with retractile testis. *J Urol.*, 147, 397A

2. Nistal, M. and Paniagua, R. (1984). Infertility in adult males with retractile testes. *Fertil. Steril.*, 41, 395

Related subjects: cryptorchidism, orchidopexy, physical examination — male infertility, scrotal temperature

RETROGRADE EJACULATION

Retrograde ejaculation is caused by impairment of the functional integrity of the bladder neck and the posterior urethra. Due to this, the posterior urethral sphincter is not closed at seminal emission. It is an uncommon cause of male infertility, at less than 1% . The condition has to be excluded in all cases of azoospermia. It can be congenital, acquired (neurogenic or traumatic) or idiopathic in origin. Common etiological factors include sequelae from traumatic paraplegia, radical lymph node dissection, diabetic neuropathy, transurethral resection of the prostate, bladder neck Y-V surgery. An initial trial of medical therapy is warranted.The agents commonly used are α-adrenergic agonists (phenylpropanolamine, ephedrine sulfate, imipramine HCl). Successful recovery of spermatozoa from urine is dependent upon an adequate medium being present in the bladder during ejaculation, this can be either urine with optimal pH and osmolarity or medium installed into the bladder prior to ejaculation. Depending on the quality of the obtained spermatozoa, either intrauterine insemination or *in vitro* fertilization is the treatment of choice.

1. Yavetz, H., Yogev, L., Hauser, R., Lessing, J.B., Paz, G. and Hommonai, Z.T. (1994). Retrograde ejaculation. A review. *Hum. Reprod.*, 9(3), 381

Related subjects: azoospermia, diabetes mellitus, medication — treatment, paraplegia, sexual function — drugs interfering, spinal cord injury

S s

SCROTAL TEMPERATURE

The temperature in the scrotum is several degrees cooler than in the abdominal cavity. Elevated intrascrotal temperature can impair spermatogenesis. Depending on the degree and the duration of the exposure, it may induce reversible oligozoospermia with spermatogenic arrest at the primary spermatocyte level or affect sperm parameters including count, morphology and motility. Frequent use of saunas, fever, varicocele, jockey underpants, occupational and environmental exposure to heat, and wheelchair-bound, spinal-cord injured men are known inducers of elevated intrascrotal temperature. The effects of hyperthermia could be studied by placing testis in a high near-inguinal position which method of artificial cryptorchidism was developed as a possible method for contraception.

1. Bedford, J.M. (1991). Effects of elevated temperature on the epididymis and testis: experimental studies. *Adv. Exp. Med. Biol.*, **286**, 19

2. Mieusset, R., Grandjean, H. and Mansat, A. (1985). Inhibiting effect of artificial cryptorchidism on spermatogenesis. *Fertil. Steril.*, **43**, 589

3. Oates, R.D. (1991). Nonsurgical treatment of infertility: specific therapy. In Lipshultz, L.I. and Howard, S.S. (eds.) *Infertility in the Male*, 2nd edn, p. 376. (St Louis: Mosby-Year Book)

Related subjects: cryptorchidism, history — male infertility, spermatogenic arrest, varicocele

SEASONAL VARIATION

Literature reporting on sperm parameters often finds a deterioration in count, motility and morphology during summer. This reduction in sperm quality could contribute to the deficit in the numbers of spring births seen in non-equatorial climates. Further analysis, however, makes it unlikely that summer heat or exposure to increased light intensity are the causative factors for this phenomenon. More likely, it relates to photoperiodicity (length of daylight), especially since serum testosterone shows a seasonal pattern, highest in winter and lowest in summer.

1. Levine, R.J., Brown, M.H., Bell, M., Shue, F., Greenberg, G.N. and Bordson, B.L. (1992). Air-conditioned environments do not prevent deterioration of human semen quality during the summer. *Fertil. Steril.*, **57**(5), 1075

2. Mallidis, C., Howard, E.J. and Baker, H.W. (1991). Variation of semen quality in normal men. *Int. J. Androl.*, 14(2), 99

Related subjects: semen analysis — normal values

SEMEN ANALYSIS, BIOCHEMICAL TESTS OF SEMINAL PLASMA

Contributions to seminal plasma are made in part by secretions from the sexual accessory glands, each with their distinct biochemical constitution. Therefore these substances (see Table 28) can be used as markers for abnormality of the glands. Markers are being expressed as quantity per ejaculate.

Table 28   The substances tested in seminal plasma as markers of abnormality

Test	Comment	Normal value
Acid phosphatase	marker of prostatic function	> 200 U/ejaculate
Carnitine	mainly of epididymal origin expensive assay	390–1830 nmol/ejaculation
Citric acid	marker of prostatic function	> 52 µmol/ejaculation
Fructose	marker of seminal vesicle function	> 13 µmol/ejaculation
α-Glucosidase	specific marker of epididymal function	> 20 mU/ejaculation
Zinc	marker of prostatic function	> 2.4 µmol/ejaculation

1. Comhaire, F.H., Vermeulen, L. and Schoonjans, F. (1987). Reassesment of the accuracy of traditional sperm characteristics and adenosine triphosphate (ATP) in the fertilizing potential of human semen *in vivo*. *Int. J. Androl.*, 10, 653

2. World Health Organization (1992). *WHO Laboratory Manual for the Examination of Human Semen and Sperm–Cervical Mucus Interaction*, 3rd edn. (Cambridge: Cambridge University Press)

Related subjects: epididymis, prostate, seminal vesicle

SEMEN ANALYSIS, BIOCHEMICAL TESTS OF SPERMATOZOA

These tests can be considered as indirect functional tests of the spermatozoa, as it measures substances derived from the spermatozoa. They are listed in Table 29.

1. Aitken, J. and Fisher, H. (1994). Reactive oxygen species generation and human spermatozoa: the balance of benefit and risk. *Bioessays*, 16(4), 259

2. Comhaire, F.H., Vermeulen, L. and Schoonjans, F. (1987). Reassessment of the accuracy of traditional sperm characteristics and adenosine triphosphate (ATP) in the fertilizing potential of human semen *in vivo*. *Int. J. Androl.*, 10, 653

Table 29   The tests used to assess the function of spermatozoa

Test	Background	Comment
Acrosin	protease enzyme from acrosome inactive form is pro-acrosin	quantitative enzymatic gelatine slide test; assessment at individual cell level
Adenosine triphosphate (ATP)	ATP is the energy source motility	marker of motility and count poor correlation with fertilizing potential
Chromatin condensation	test of functional and structural status since inactive chromatin is highly condensed	aniline blue acridine orange fluorescence; can be used with flow cytometry
Creatine kinase	high levels of creatine kinase are related to retained cytoplasm; immaturity	predictor of fertilizing capacity
Hyaluronidase	involved in sperm penetration of cumulus mass; also located in acrosome	
Reactive oxygen species	reactive oxygen species or free radicals can be generated by leukocytes and by certain sub-populations of spermatozoa because of retained cytoplasm	impaired fertilizing capacity

3. Evenson, D.P., Jost, L., Baer, R.K., Turner, T.W. and Schrader, S.M. (1991). Individuality of DNA denaturation patterns in human sperm as measured by the sperm chromatinstructure assay. *Reprod. Toxicol.*, 5, 115

4. Huszar, G. and Vigue, L. (1993). Incomplete development of human spermatozoa is associated with increased creatin phosphokinase concentration and abnormal head morphology. *Mol. Reprod. Dev.*, 34(30), 292

5. Kennedy, W.P., Kaminski, J.M., van der Ven, H.H., Jeyendran, R.S., Reid, D.S., Blackwell, J., Bielfeld, P. and Zaneveld, L.J.D. (1989). A simple, clinical assay to evaluate the acrosin activity of human spermatozoa. *J. Androl.*, 10, 221

6. Polakoski, K.L. and Zaneveld, L.J.D. (1977). Biochemical examination of the human ejaculate. In Hafez, E.S.E. (ed.) *Techniques of Human Andrology*. (Amsterdam: Elsevier/North Holland)

Related subjects: acrosome reaction, creatine kinase, motility, oxygen — reactive species, sperm function test

SEMEN ANALYSIS, COLLECTION OF SAMPLE

To ensure optimal and standardized conditions for delivery of a sample to the andrology laboratory for analysis the following is required:

(1) The container has to be delivered to the laboratory with the patient's name, date and time of collection;

(2) A prescribed period of abstinence prior to the collection must have occurred;

(3) The sample has to be produced by direct masturbation into the container (the use of condoms or coitus interruptus is not acceptable);

(4) The sample has to be delivered within 60 minutes of production; and

(6) A non-toxic, sterile and wide container is to be used for collection.

Related subjects: asthenozoospermia, semen analysis — normal values

SEMEN ANALYSIS, NORMAL VALUES (Table 30)

The purest definition of a normal semen sample would be that, if the sample had been inseminated into a fertile female at coitus, it would have resulted in a pregnancy. This definition, however, takes into account both the fertilizing capacity of the semen and the fertility of the female. When trying to predict fertility based on data obtained by visual measures of semen analysis, it should be realized that these data are prone to be inaccurate: high coefficients of variation have been reported for the same and between different technicians, as well as between different laboratories, for count, morphology and motility. So-called normal values always represent the lower end of normality and distributions of most biological variables gradually show transition from normal to subnormal and pathological. Regional differences in normality exist. As long as clearly defined laboratory standardization has not been reached and each laboratory has to deal with a possible different population, each laboratory should ideally determine its own range of normal values. The literature is controversial as to how many samples have to be analyzed before a reliable estimation of a patient's fertility potential can be made. Several authors agree that if a first sample is fully classified as normal according to the laboratory standards, no further analysis is needed. However, if the result of the analysis is abnormal a second or even a third sample should be obtained within 3 months.

The result of a semen analysis, normal or abnormal, has to be interpreted in conjunction with the personal background information of the involved individual. It is well known that many obvious factors may influence the result of a semen analysis. The following factors are possible contributors to variation:

(1) Abstinence period;

(2) Occupational hazards;

(3) Previous illness;

(4) Seasonal influences; and

(5) Stress;

(6) Toxins such as smoking or alcohol.

Table 30 The values established as normal by the World Health Organization in 1992

Parameter	World Health Organization 1992
Volume	> 2.0 ml
pH	7.2–8.0
Concentration	> 20 × 10⁶/ml
Total count	> 40 × 10⁶/ml
Motility	> 50% (rapid, slow or sluggish progressive)
Motility	> 25% (rapid progressive)
Morphology	> 30% normal
Vitality	> 75% live
Leukocytes	< 1.0 × 10⁶/ml
Immunobead test	< 20% sperm with beads
Mixed agglutination reaction (MAR) test	< 10% sperm with RBC

1. Carlsen, E., Giwercman, A., Keiding, N. and Skakkebaek, N.E. (1992). Evidence for decreasing sperm quality of semen during the past 50 years. *Br. Med. J.*, **305**, 609

2. Menkveld, R. and Kruger, T.F. (1990). Basic semen analysis. In Acosta, A.A. (ed.) *Human Spermatozoa in Assisted Reproduction.* (Baltimore: Williams and Wilkins)

3. Mortimer, D. (1994). Semen analysis. In Mortimer, D. (ed.) *Practical Laboratory Andrology.* (Oxford: Oxford University Press)

4. Poland, M.L., Moghissi, K.S., Giblin, P.T., Ager, J.W. and Olson, J.M. (1985). Variation of semen measure within normal men. *Fertil. Steril.*, **44**, 396

5. World Health Organization (1992). *WHO Laboratory Manual for the Examination of Human Semen and Sperm–Cervical Mucus Interaction,* 3rd edn. (Cambridge: Cambridge University Press)

Related subjects: abstinence period, aging, history — male infertility, occupational hazards, semen analysis — predictive value, stress

SEMEN ANALYSIS, PHYSICAL PROPERTIES (Table 31)

Table 31   The physical properties of semen analysis

Parameter	Comment
Coagulation	quick coagulation, 10–15 minutes after ejaculation by proteinkinase from seminal vesicle
Liquefaction	normal within 30 minutes, by fibrinolysin from prostate, fibrinogenase and aminopeptidase
Viscosity	arbitrary measurement by length of thread of semen
Color	when normal it is white-gray-yellowish; when contaminated it is yellow (urine) or pink to red (blood)
Opacity	opalescent
Odor	subjective and variable
pH	7.2–8.2 normal range, altered in case of infections of prostate or seminal vesicle
Volume	normal 2.0–6.0 ml
Buffering capacity	41.1 ± Slyke

1. Wolters-Everhardt, E., Dony, J.M., Lemmens, W.A., Doesburg, W.H. and DePont, J.J. (1986). Buffering capacity of human semen. *Fertil. Steril.*, 46(1), 114

2. World Health Organization (1992). *WHO Laboratory Manual for the Examination of Human Semen and Sperm–Cervical Mucus Interaction*, 3rd edn. (Cambridge: Cambridge University Press)

Related subjects: prostate, semen analysis — processing of sample, seminal vesicle

SEMEN ANALYSIS, PREDICTIVE VALUE

Single parameters of human semen analysis or the number of abnormal parameters cannot accurately distinguish between fertile or infertile men. The qualitative aspects of spermiogenesis (morphology, motility and vitality) are related to each other, but also to the quantitative apect of spermatogenesis (i.e. the numbers of spermatozoa produced). The predictive value of semen analysis is low when the duration of the infertility is short. Probably the best predictive value for pregnancy (of at about 50%) can be obtained by multivariate discriminant analysis of volume, count, per cent motility plus normal morphology. When computer-aided semen analysis is included, the literature reports that some parameters like amplitude of lateral head displacement can improve the discriminatory power of semen analysis. Reasons for poor predictive value of semen analysis are variations in measurement (intra- and interobserver) and deficient correlation of semen analysis with fertility.

1. Aitken, R.J., Best, F.S.M., Warner, P. and Templeton, A. (1984). A prospective study of the relationship between semen quality and fertility in cases of unexplained infertility. *J. Androl.*, 5, 297

2. Bartoov, B., Eltes, F., Pansky, M., Lederman, H., Caspi, E. and Soffer, Y. (1993). Estimating fertility potential via semen analysis data. *Hum. Reprod.*, 8(1), 65

3. Bielsa, M.A., Andolz, P., Gris, P.M., Martinez, P. and Egoscue, J. (1994). Which semen parameters have a predictive value for pregnancy in infertile couples? *Hum. Reprod.*, 9, 1887

4. Dunphy, B.C., Neal, L.M. and Cooke, I.D. (1989). The clinical value of conventional semen analysis. *Fertil. Steril.*, 51, 324

5. Wichmann, L., Isola, J. and Tuohimaa, P. (1994). Prognostic variables in predicting pregnancy. A prospective follow up study of 907 couples with an infertility problem. *Hum. Reprod.*, 9(6), 1102

Related subjects: computer-aided semen analysis, statistics

SEMEN ANALYSIS, PROCESSING OF SAMPLE (Figure 29)

1. World Health Organization (1992). *WHO laboratory Manual for the Examination of Human Semen and Sperm–Cervical Mucus Interaction*, 3rd edn. (Cambridge: Cambridge University Press)

Related subjects: computer aided semen analysis, morphology — normal — abnormal, motility, semen analysis — normal values, semen analysis — biochemical test seminal plasma and spermatozoa

SEMINAL PLASMA MOTILITY INHIBITOR (SPMI)

Human seminal plasma contains a protein that inhibits motility of spermatozoa. This seminal plasma motility inhibitor is exclusively derived from the seminal vesicles. The levels of SPMI in seminal plasma are too low to affect motility of normal spermatozoa. A few minutes after ejaculation most of the SPMI present in the seminal vesicle is inactivated. The substance may be involved in the immobilization of spermatozoa of poorer quality.

1. Iwamoto, T. and Gagnon, C. (1988). A human seminal plasma protein blocks the motility of human spermatozoa. *J. Urol.*, 140, 1045

Related subjects: motility, semen analysis — collection of sample, seminal vesicle

SEMINAL VESICLE

The seminal vesicle is formed by a paired convoluted tube of 5–6 cm in length and a diameter of 3–4 mm. It is located on the dorsal surface of the bladder. Its opening is located just below the ampulla of the ductus deferens. It has a multiglandular function and exclusively secretes fructose and prostaglandins. It contributes 70% to the ejaculate volume and delivers the last fraction of spermatozoa. One ejaculate almost completely depletes the content of the seminal vesicle. Congenital absence of the vas deferens is

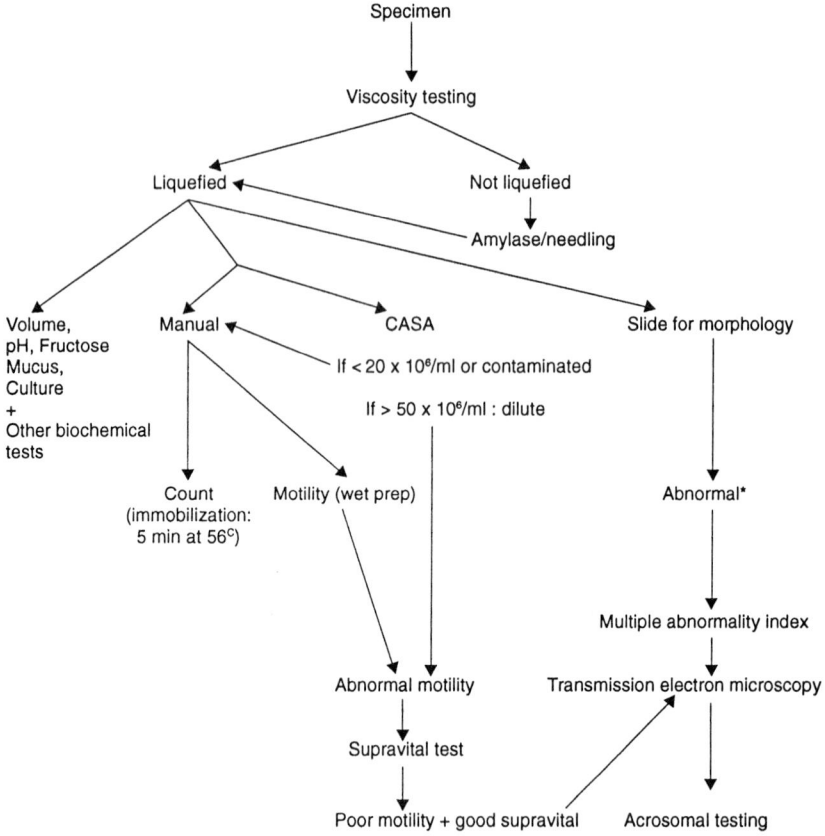

Figure 29 A flow chart providing guidelines on the processing of a sample during semen analysis

*abnormal morphology according to WHO/strict criteria or depending on monovariate morphological abnormalities (e.g. high percentage of globospermia, more than 10% immature cells or more than 10% of coiled tails – poor handling prior to analysis ?)

associated with agenesis of the seminal vesicle, since both structures have the same embryonic origin.

1. Mortimer, D. (1994). *Practical Laboratory Andrology.* (Oxford: Oxford University Press)

Related subjects: anatomy, ejaculate — composition, semen analysis — biochemical test of seminal plasma

SERTOLI CELL

The Sertoli cells are one of the two major cell components of the seminiferous tubules. They rest on the basal lamina and are connected to each other by tight junctions. Together with the myoid cells they form the blood–testis barrier. The Sertoli cells are assumed to have the following functions:

(1) Sustenance of the germ cells. They metabolize (e.g. glucose into lactate and pyruvate) and synthesize transferrin necessary for iron delivery to the cells.

(2) Maintenance of the blood–testis barrier and physical support for the germ cells as each Sertoli cell is, on average, in contact with 47 germ cells.

(3) Production of specific proteins such as androgen binding protein and inhibin.

(4) Synthesis of estradiol through aromatization of androgens.

(5) Principal site of follicle stimulating hormone and testosterone action.

1. Veldhuis, J. (1991). The hypothalamic–pituitary–testicular axis. In Yen, S.S.C. and Jaffe, R.B. (eds.) *Reproductive Endocrinology*, 3rd edn. (Philadelphia: W.B.Saunders)

Related subjects: androgen binding protein, blood–testis barrier, endocrinology

SERTOLI CELL-ONLY SYNDROME

The syndrome is characterized by loss of germ cells with relative preservation of the Leydig cells. Follicle stimulating hormone levels are elevated, luteinizing hormone levels may vary from normal to high. Clinically diminished testicular volume, soft testes and azoospermia are found. The diagnosis requires testicular biopsy. It is probably the end stage of a condition resulting from different pathological processes, although histopathology obtained from needle aspiration or testicular biopsy is not necessarily representative of the entire testis. Hence, it is possible that spermatozoa are obtained from testis previously reported to show atrophy or Sertoli cell-only.

1. Silber, S.J., van Steiteghem, A.C. and Devroey, P. (1995). Sertoli cell revisited. *Hum. Reprod.*, **10**(5), 1031

2. Yemini, M., Vanderzwalmen, P., Mukaida, T., Schoengold, S. and Birkenfeld, A. (1995). Intracytoplasmic sperm injection, fertilization and embryo transfer after retrieval of spermatozoa by testicular biopsy from an azoospermic male with testicular tubular atrophy. *Fertil Steril.*, **63**(5), 1118

Related subjects: azoospermia, hypergonadotropic hypogonadism, testicular biopsy — histopathology

SEX SELECTION

In the past attempts have been made to preselect the sex of a child before conception in many different ways (Table 32).

None of the methods showed significantly different figures for the the desired sex or the results could not be reproduced by others. A recent improvement in this regard has been made by the application of stain to the spermatozoa followed by flow cytometry to segregate X- and Y-bearing

Table 32   The different methods used to preselect the sex of a child

Method	Sex with increased chance
Period of abstinence prior to ovulation	abstinence > 3 days: male
Cooling down of scrotum	male
Positioning and depth of penetration	deep: male
Timing of coitus to ovulation	close: male
Female and/or male orgasm	female orgasm: male
Modification of the pH of the cervical mucus by vaginal douches or diets	alkaline: male
Ovulation drugs such as clomiphene or human menopausal gonadotropin	female
Insemination with fresh or frozen/thawed semen	fresh: male
Separation of the larger and slower moving X chromosome bearing sperm (4% more DNA) from the faster Y chromosome-bearing sperm	Sephadex: female Albumin gradient: male

spermatozoa based on their difference in the amount of DNA. This method results in separation for X spermatozoa of 80–90% and for Y-bearing spermatozoa of 65–70%.

1. Edwards, R.G. and Beard, H.K. (1995). Sexing human spermatozoa to control sex ratios at birth is now a reality. *Mol. Hum. Reprod.*, 1, 977

2. Levinson, G., Keyvanfar, K. and Wu, J.C. (1995). DNA-based X-enriched sperm separation as an adjunct to preimplantation genetic testing for the prevention of X-linked disease. *Mol. Hum. Reprod.*, 1, 979

3. Shettles *et al.* (1984). How to Choose the Sex of Your Baby, p. 109. (Garden City, Doubleday)

4. Windsor, D.P., Evans, G. and White, I.G. (1993). Sex predetermination by separation of X and Y chromosome-bearing sperm: a review. *Reprod. Fertil. Dev.*, 5(2), 155

5. Zarutski, P.W., Muller, C.H., Magone, M. and Soules, M.R. (1989). The clinical relevance of sex selection techniques. *Fertil. Steril.*, 52(6), 891

Related subjects: flow cytometry, sperm preparation

SEXUAL DYSFUNCTION (Table 33)

1. Montague, D.K. (1988). *Disorders of Male Sexual Function.* (Chicago: Year Book Medical Publishers)

Related subjects: androgen therapy, anejaculation, azoospermia, diabetes mellitus, hyperprolactinemia, retrograde ejaculation, sexual function — drugs interfering, sexual function — terminology

Table 33   The different types of sexual dysfunction

	Type	*Comment*
Libido	hypoactive desire	libido that is experienced as being abnormal low, either by the patient, the partner or both
	hyperactive desire	libido felt as abnormally high
Erectile dysfunction	prepenile	psychogenic, organic (normal penile anatomy)
	penile	organic (abnormal penile anatomy)
	priapism	only corpora cavernosa erect (abnormal, prolonged, painful erection, not associated with continuous sexual stimulation)
Ejaculatory dysfunction	premature	functional (ejaculation sooner than desired, before, during or after intromission)
	retarded	psychogenic (inability to have an orgasm during voluntary sexual activity)
	orgasm without apparent ejaculation	retrograde (into the bladder), failure of seminal emission (semen not deposited into posterior urethra), aspermia (failure of semen and seminal fluid)
	anorgasmia	organic
Sensory disturbances		absent/impaired sensation during any phase of sexual activity
	pain	

SEXUAL FUNCTION, TERMINOLOGY

Terminology used in describing male sexual (dys)functions is listed in Table 34.

1. Montague, D.K. (1988). *Disorders of Male Sexual Function.* (Chicago: Year Book Medical Publishers)

Related subjects: sexual dysfunction, sexual function — drugs interfering

Table 34   The terms used when discussing male sexual function

Term	Comment
Ejaculation	forcible expulsion of semen
Emission	deposition of semen into the posterior (prostatic) urethra
Erection	starting from the flaccid state, the penis becomes tumescent (increase in size) and then develops rigidity
Flaccid	non-erect penis
Intromission	introduction of the erect penis into a body cavity
Latency, refractory period	the time period between one ejaculation and the ability to obtain another erection (erectile latency) or ejaculation (ejaculatory latency)
Libido	the urge or drive to initiate sexual activity
Orgasm	the sensory experience of a sudden relief of sexual tension
Rigidity	increase in intracorporeal pressure that allows force to be directed through the glans penis to the long axis of the penis without a sudden collapse of the penis
Thrusting	in and out movements of the usually erect penis within a body cavity
Tumescence	increase in length and circumference of the penis

SEXUAL FUNCTION, DRUGS INTERFERING WITH NORMAL MALE

These are listed and discussed in Tables 35, 36 and 37.

1. Olin, B.R. (ed.) *Drug, Facts and Comparisons.* (St Louis: Mosby Year Book)

2. Dukes, M.N.G. (ed.) (1988). *Meyler's Side Effects of Drugs. An Encyclopedia of Adverse Reactions and Interactions.* (Amsterdam : Elsevier)

3. Gilbert, B.R. (1995). Transurethral resection for ejaculatory duct obstruction. In Goldstein, M. (ed.) *Surgery for Male Infertility.* (Philadelphia: W.B. Saunders)

Related subjects: drug abuse, history — male infertility, retrograde ejaculation, sexual dysfunction

Table 35   Drugs that effect ejaculation

Clomipramine	tricyclic antidepressant	spontaneous orgasm; delay or abolition of ejaculation
Clonidine	central acting antiadrenergic; antihypertensive	retrograde ejaculation
Disopyramide	antiarrhythmic agent; ventricular tachycardia	erectile impotence
Flecainide	antiarrhythmic agent; paroxysmal atrial flutter, ventricular arrhythmia	erectile impotence
Guanethidine	peripheral acting antiadrenergic; antihypertensive	failure of ejaculation
MAO inhibitors	increase monoamine concentration; antidepressant, antiparkinson	delayed ejaculation; difficulty in achieving orgasm
Naproxen	prostaglandin synthetase inhibitor	impotence – failure of ejaculation
Neuroleptics	anticholinergic activity	erectile and ejaculatory dysfunction; priapism; retrograde ejaculation; spontaneous ejaculation
Phenoxybenzamine	α-adrenergic receptor blocker; pheochromocytoma	inhibition of ejaculation
Thioridazine	phenothiazine; antipsychotic	impotence; retrograde ejaculation; spontaneous ejaculation
Tolazoline	peripheral vasodilator; antihypertensive	ejaculation failure
Trazodone	MAO inhibitor; antidepressant	inhibition of ejaculation; priapism
Tricyclic antidepressants	due to anticholinergic action	loss of erectile function; delayed ejaculation; delayed orgasm
Warfarin		priapism

MAO = monoamine oxidase

Table 36 Drugs that effect potence

Acetazolamide	non-bacteriostatic sulfonamide inhibiting carbonic anhydase; glaucoma, diuretic	loss of libido; impotence
Anticonvulsants	phenytoin; primidone; phenobarbital	decreased libido; impotence
β-blockers		impotence
Cimetidine	histamine H_2 antagonist; anti-ulcer	impotence
Clofibrate	antihyperlipidemic	impotence
Clomipramine	tricyclic antidepressant	sexual arousal
Clonidine	central acting antiadrenergic; antihypertensive	impotence
Fenfluramine	sympathimemetic amine; anorectic agent	impotence
Guanethidine	peripheral acting antiadrenergic; antihypertensive	impotence
Hydralazine	vasodilator; antihypertensive	impotence
Hydroxyprogesterone caproate	long-acting progestin; benign prostatic hyperplasia	impotence
MAO inhibitors	antidepressant; antiparkinson	relative impotence
Methyldopa	antiadrenergic; antihypertensive	impotence
Naproxen	prostaglandin synthetase inhibitor	impotence
Prazosin	peripheral acting; antiadrenergic antihypertensive	impotence
Propafenone	antiarrhythmic agent; ventricular arrhythmia	impotence
Spironolactone	K sparing diuretic; aldosterone antagonist; hyperaldosteronism	loss of libido; impotence
Thiazide diuretics	increase excretion of sodium and chloride; antihypertensives	impotence?
Tricyclic antidepressants	due to anticholinergic action	impotence

MAO = monoamine oxidase

Table 37 Drugs that effect libido

Amphetamines	sympathomimetic; narcolepsy; obesity; abuse	from unchanged to decreased, mixed or heightened libido
Anticonvulsants	phenytoin; primidone; phenobarbital	decreased sexual activity
β-adrenoceptor blockers	hypertension; angina pectoris; arrhythmia	decreased sexual activity
Colchicine	antigout agent	progressive decrease in libido
Levodopa	metabolic precursor of dopamine; parkinsonism	increase in libido
Lithium	effects neurotransmitter metabolism; antimanic agent	decrease in libido
Mazindol	non-amphetaminic anorectic; obesity	increase in libido
Neuroleptics	anticholinergic activity	decrease in libido; changes in quality orgasm
Spironolactone	K sparing diuretic; aldosterone antagonist; hyperaldosteronism	loss of libido
Tricyclic antidepressants	due to anticholinergic action	both increase and decrease in libido reported

SEXUALLY TRANSMITTED DISEASES, RELATION TO MALE INFERTILITY

The consequences of AIDS for male infertility are discussed under a separate heading. The incidence of sexually transmitted diseases like gonorrhea, syphylis and *Chlamydia* is steadily increasing. There is an established causal relationship between sexually transmitted diseases and male infertility (see Table 38). Therefore, sequelae like leukocytospermia, obstruction of the ejaculatory ducts and testicular atrophy are likely to increase as well. There is controversy about the consequences of bacteriospermia in male fertility. One of the main reasons for this is the fact that diagnostic criteria for bacteriospermia are controversial.

Infected semen may be diagnosed if at least two of the following features are present:

(1) History of urogenital infection or abnormal prostate on palpation;

(2) Abnormal secretion after prostatic massage;

Table 38   Relation of sexually transmitted disease to male infertility

Micro-organism	Relation to male infertility
Neisseria gonorrheae	proven causative
Candida albicans	none
Chlamydia trachomatis	controversial
Trichomonas vaginalis	only *in vitro* data suggestive
Mycoplasma hominis	controversial
Ureaplasma urealyticum	controversial
Viruses (herpes, cytomegaly)	few data reported

(3) Greater than 1000 abnormal bacteria/ml in 1:2 diluted semen; and

(4) Greater than 1 000 000 leukocytes/ml ejaculate.

An increased number of seminal leukocytes itself is therefore not indicative of infection. Apart from the symptoms above, infection should be suspected when sperm motility is impaired, even in the absence of an increase in leukocytes. The normal male urethra is colonized by *Staphylococcus, Streptococcus* and diphtheroids. In addition, *Mycoplasma hominis* (30%) and *Ureaplasma urealyticum* (50%) have been documented in semen from normal men.

1.   Moskowitz, M.O. and Mellinger, B.C. (1992). Sexually transmitted diseases and their relation to male infertility. In Mellinger, B.C. and Smith, A.D. (eds.) Sexually transmitted diseases. *Urol. Clin. N. Am.*, **19**(1), 35

Related subjects: acquired immune deficiency syndrome, candidiasis, *Chlamydia*, culture of semen, gonococcal, human immune deficiency, virus infection, leukocytospermia, mycoplasma, syphilis, *Ureaplasma*

SICKLE CELL DISEASE

Sickle cell disease is an autosomal recessive disorder, where the gene for abnormal globin S is located on chromosome 11. It is thought that sickle cell disease may cause vaso-occlusion due to sludged sickle cells, with resulting hypoxia and infarction of areas important for male reproductive function such as the hypothalamus (low luteinizing hormone [LH], follicle stimulating hormone [FSH] and testosterone) or the testes (high FSH and LH with low testosterone) or combination thereof. In addition, vitamin or mineral (zinc) deficiencies are reported as being associated with infertility in sickle cell disease. Moreover, sickle cell disease is a risk factor for the development of priapism. With increase of age these abnormalities ameliorate.

1.   Landfeld, S.C., Schambelan, M. and Kaplan, S.L. (1983). Clomiphene responsive hypogonadism in sickle cell anemia. *Ann. Int. Med.*, **99**, 480

2. Modebe, O. and Uchechukwu, O.E. (1995). Effect of age on testicular function in adult males with sickle cell anemia. *Fertil. Steril.*, 63(4), 907

3. Prasad, A.S., Abbasi, A.A. and Rabani, P. (1981). Effect of zinc supplementation on serum testosterone level in adult male sickle cell anemia subjects. *Am. J. Hematol.*, 10, 119

Related subjects: hypergonadotropic hypogonadism, hypogonadotropic hypogonadism, nutritional deficiencies, spermatogenic arrest, zinc

SIMS–HUHNER TEST

Alternative name for postcoital test, after the gynecologists who originally described the test.

1. Huhner, M. (1921). Methods of examining for spermatozoa in the diagnosis and treatment of sterility. *Int. J. Surg.*, 34, 91

2. Sims, J.M. (1869). On the microscope as an aid in the diagnosis and treatment of sterility. *N.Y. Med. Bull.*, 8, 393

Related subjects: postcoital test

SINGLE GENE DEFECTS

With the rapidly increasing knowledge in the field of molecular biology, the understanding of genetic disease as the cause of various forms of male infertility has been elucidated. Defects can be classified as numerical or structural chromosomal anomalies, as defects in which multiple genes are involved or as so-called single-gene defects. Multiple gene (or polygene) defects refer to a group of genes that together control detectable phenotypical properties. A gene is described as a defined hereditary unit of DNA that occupies a specific position within a chromosome and determines the specific structure of a peptide chain. Already, many forms of single gene defects related to male infertility have been identified (Table 39).

1. Fauser, B.C.J.M. and Hsueh, A.J.W. (1995). Genetic basis of human reproductive endocrine disorders. *Hum. Reprod.*, 10(4), 826

Related subjects: androgen insensitivity, congenital adrenal hyperplasia, hypergonadotropic hypogonadism, hypogonadotropic hypogonadism, Kallmann's syndrome, testicular feminization

SPERMATOCELE

A spermatocele is a distension of the epididymis, usually occurring in the caput. The incidence increases with age. Therapy is usually not necessary, since they are painless and do not cause obstruction.

1. Goldstein, M. (1995). Surgery of the epididymis. In Goldstein, M. (ed.) *Surgery for Male Infertility.* (Philadelphia: W. B. Saunders)

Related subjects: epididymis, hydrocele, physical examination

Table 39 The single gene defects related to male infertility

Level of abnormally	Disorder	Located inheritance	Incidence	LH	FSH	Steroids	Clinical presentation
GnRH	Kallmann	X or autosomal	1:10 000	low	low	low T	hypogonadism
Gonadotropins	abnormal LH	chromosome 19	sporadic	high	N	low T	hypogonadism
Gonadal steroids	3β-OH steroid dehydrogenase	chromosome 1	sporadic	high	high	low T; high adrenal androgens	male pseudo-hermaphroditism to hypogonadism
Gonadal steroids	17α-hydroxylase	chromosome 10	sporadic	high	high	low T	hypogonadism
Adrenal steroids	21-hydroxylase	chromosome 6 autosomal recessive	1:10 000	N to low	N to low	high T	abnormal spermatogenesis
Androgen	androgen	X linked	1:100 000	high	high	low T	male pseudo-hermaphroditism to subfertile male

LH = luteinizing hormone; FSH = follicle stimulating hormone; GnRH = gonadotropin releasing hormone, T = testosterone

SPERMATOCELE, ALLOPLASTIC

In patients with congenital absence of the vasa deferentia, a receptacle can be implanted onto the epididymis. The method was first described by Schoysmans, using vein grafts. Because of the poor results, silicone and Gore-Tex are now generally employed. The best pregnancy rates published do not exceed 8% of couples. No pregnancies have been reported when motility of the spermatozoa obtained during operation is less than 20%. Recently, improved results have been obtained by application of *in vitro* fertilization and micromanipulation to spermatozoa obtained by this method: a fertilization percentage of 48%, and a pregnancy rate of 14%, are reported.

1. Schoysman, R. (1968). La creation d'une spermatocele artificielle dans les agenesies du canal deferent. *Bull. Soc. Belg. Gynecol. Obstet.*, 38, 317

2. Wagenknecht, L.V., Leidenberger, F.A. and Schutte, B. (1978). Clinical experience with an alloplastic spermatocele. *Andrologia*, 10, 417

3. Wagenknecht, L.V. (1995). Alloplastic spermatocele. In Goldstein, M. (ed.) *Surgery of Male Infertility*. (Philadelphia: W.B. Saunders)

Related subjects: azoospermia, congenital absence vas deferens, cystic fibrosis, microepididymal sperm aspiration, percutaneous epididymal sperm aspiration, spermatocele — autogenous

SPERMATOCELE, AUTOGENOUS

A recently described microsurgical technique, involving marsupialization of an epididymal tubule to the visceral layer of the tunica vaginalis, thus creating an autogenous sperm reservoir. The first experiences showed successful sperm aspiration in 30% of cases.

1. Moni, V.N. and Lalitha, P.A.(1992). Moni's window operation: a new surgical technique to create a sperm reservoir in congenital vasal agenesis. *J. Urol.*, 148, 843

Related subjects: azoospermia, congenital absence of vas deferens, cystic fibrosis, microepididymal sperm aspiration, percutaneous epididymal sperm aspiration, spermatocele — alloplastic

SPERMATOGENESIS

The spermatogonium is a cell capable of either undergoing mitotic division or of entering the meiotic events giving rise to a primary spermatocyte. Spermatogenesis is the process by which a spermatogonial stem cell undergoes meiotic divisions, proliferates and ultimately is transformed into free spermatozoa. This process requires about 64 days in the human and is described in Table 40 (see also Figure 30).

Ultimately, every diploid spermatogonium entering the meiotic sequence of events will result in the formation of four haploid spermatozoa. Spermatogenesis takes place in the seminiferous tubules from the basal lamina towards the lumen. The lateral cytoplasmic extensions of the Sertoli cells act

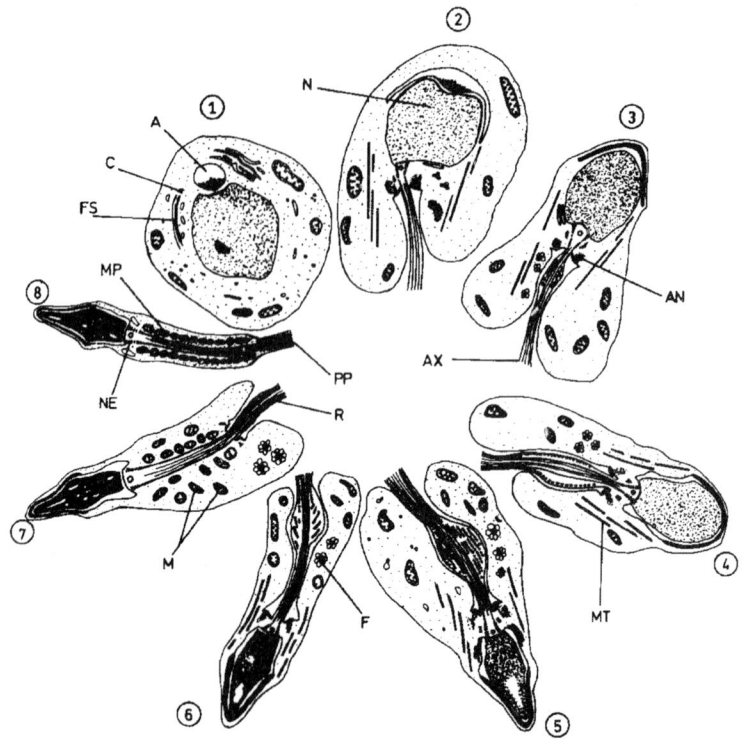

Figure 30 Spermatogenesis, showing the condensation of the nucleus, formation of the acrosome, formation of the axoneme, the fibrous sheath, and the Adaptele association of mitochondria in the midpiece. N = nucleus, A = acrosome, AX = axoneme, R = fibrous sheath, M = mitochondria, C = Centriole, FS = fibrous sheath, MT = microtubules, AN = anulus, NE = neck, MP = midpiece, PP = principle piece, F = flagellum. (From Kelly, D. E. Wood, R. L. , Enders, A. Co. (eds): Bailey's Textbook of Microscopic Anatomy, 18th edn. Baltimore: Williams & Wilkins, 1984, p. 697.)

as escalators in this movement. This movement forms an upward narrowing helix which converges with other helices, so that when a tubule is sectioned, different stages of spermatogenesis can be seen.

Related subjects: anatomy, Sertoli cell

SPERMATOGENIC ARREST

Spermatogenic arrest is the cessation of germ cell differentiation from spermatogonium to spermatozoon. This event may occur at any stage in the development of the spermatozoa, depending on the etiology. Partial arrest leads to oligozoospermia, complete arrest to azoospermia. The diagnosis is made by testicular biopsy. Spermatogenic arrest has to be differentiated from hypospermatogenesis, where all stages of spermatogenesis are represented in

Table 40 The spermatogenesis process

Name	*Type*	*Age*	*Position*	*Genetic*	*Characteristics*
Spermatogonia	primordial germ cell	< birth	basal lamina	mitosis diploid	large, light stain,
	fetal	< 6 years	"	"	large, disperse chromatin
	transitional	< 6 years	"	"	less disperse chromatin
	type Ap	> birth– adult	"	"	round, pale, peripheral nucleolus
	type Ad	> birth– adult	"	"	dark, chromatin, resting stem cell
	type Al		"	"	more flat and elongated
	type Ac		"	"	cloudy chromatin variant Ap
	type B	> 4 years	"	"	smaller, looser from basal lamina
Spermatocytes	primary		immediate	DNA doubling tetraploid preleptotene	
	primary		"	leptotene	
	primary		"	zygotene	
	primary		"	pachytene	
	primary		"	1st meiosis diplotene	
	secondary		adluminal	diploid second meiosis	
Spermatids	Golgi phase Sa1		adluminal	haploid	
	Golgi phase Sa2		"	"	
	cap phase Sb1		"	"	
	cap phase Sb2		"	"	
	acrosome phase Sc1		adluminal	haploid	
	acrosome phase Sd2		"	"	
	maturation phase Sd1		"	"	
	maturation phase Sd2		"	"	
Spermatozoon			seminiferous tubule	"	

the testicular biopsy, but in decreased numbers. In case of arrest the presence of different cells halts at the level of cessation. Arrest also has to be distinguished from obstruction by testicular biopsy, since some patients with spermatogenic arrest have normal values for gonadotropic hormones. The literature reports an incidence of 5–30% for spermatogenic arrest in cases with severe oligozoospermia or azoospermia. Several levels of arrest can be distinguished:

(1) Spermatogonial level: observed after radiation, alkylating cytostatic drugs, use of gonadotropin releasing hormone agonists;

(2) Primary spermatocyte level: vitamin A deficiency, liver and renal disease, hyperthermia; and

(3) Spermatid level: seen after gonadotropin deficiency, diabetes.

Some causes show a specific level of spermatogenic arrest as mentioned above, but different levels are reported for others, such as for varicocele, in which spermatogenic arrest can occur at the primary spermatocyte and the spermatid level (Table 41).

Table 41   Primary and secondary spermatogenic arrest

Primary	Chromosomal (somatic cell) Chromosomal (germ cell)	XXY, XYY, trisomy, translocation
Secondary	Testicular	cryptorchidism; torsion; varicocele
	Endocrine	Hypogonadism; adrenal hyperplasia; hyperprolactinemia; androgen insensitivity
	Iatrogenic	radiation; cytostatics; gonadotropin releasing hormone agonist; certain antibiotics
	Metabolic	vitamin A and zinc deficiency; liver/ renal disease; sickle cell disease
	Temperature	febrile illness, sauna

1.   Martin-du-Pan, R.C. and Campana, A. (1993). Physiopathology of spermatogenic arrest. *Fertil. Steril.*, 60(6), 937

Related subjects: antibiotics, chemotherapy, chromosomal abnormalities, cryptorchidism, history — male infertility, hypergonadotropic hypogonadism, hypogonadotropic hypogonadism, liver disease, nutritional deficiencies, radiation exposure, renal failure, sickle cell disease, testicular biopsy — histopathology, torsion – testis, varicocele, zinc

SPERM–CERVICAL MUCUS CONTACT TEST (SCMC)

This is a slide test where spermatozoa and cervical mucus are mixed to detect the presence of any sperm immobilizing antibodies in either the cervical mucus or the seminal plasma. Cross-testing using donor semen and donor mucus can be performed in case of a positive result.

1. Kremer, J. and Jager, S. (1978). The sperm–cervical mucus contact test: a preliminary report. *Fertil. Steril.*, 27, 335

Related subjects: Kremer test, Kurzrok–Miller test

SPERM COLLECTION TECHNIQUES

In azoospermia with some degree of spermatogenesis, spermatozoa can be collected from patients with different problems. Depending on the indication for which the sperm collection is performed (see Table 42), the quality and the quantity of the spermatozoa obtained, further fertility management has to be planned. This may include intracervical or intrauterine insemination, the latter possibly in combination with ovarian hyperstimulation. With poorer spermatozoa *in vitro* fertilization and even intracytoplasmic sperm injection may have to be included. A pivotal part is cryopreservation of the

Table 42   The indications for the different sperm collection techniques

Type of azoospermia	Disease	Sperm collection technique
Disconnective	congenital absence vas deferens obstruction: (a) congenital, (b) infectious, or (c) iatrogenic	spermatocele: (a) alloplastic, or (b) autogenous microsurgical epidydimal sperm aspiration testicular sperm aspiration
Anejaculation	spinal cord injury multiple sclerosis diabetes mellitus anorgasm	medical stimulation: (a) vibratory, or (b) electro-ejaculation surgical: (a) vas deferens sperm aspiration, (b) microsurgical epididymal sperm aspiration, (c) percutaneous epididymal sperm aspiration, or (d) testicular sperm aspiration
Impaired spermatogenesis	Sertoli cell syndrome testicular atrophy spermatogenic arrest	testicular sperm aspiration testicular exploration and sperm extraction

spermatozoa which are not for immediate use, since freezing/thawing techniques are successfully combined with *in vitro* fertilization and intracytoplasmic sperm injection.

1. Jow, W.W., Steckel, J., Schlegel, P.N., Magid, M.S. and Goldstein, M. (1993). Motile sperm in human testis biopsy specimens. *J. Androl.*, 14, 194

2. Palermo, G., Joris, H., Devroey, P. and van Steirteghem, A.C. (1992). Pregnancies after intracytoplasmic sperm injection of single spermatozoon into an oocyte. *Lancet*, 340, 17

3. Schlegel, P.N., Berkeley, A.S. and Goldstein, M. (1994). Epididymal micropuncture with *in vitro* fertilization and oocyte micromanipulation for the treatment of unreconstructable obstructive azoospermia. *Fertil. Steril.*, 61, 895

4. Silber, S.J., van Steirteghem, A.C., Liu, J., Nagy, Z., Tournaye, H. and Devroey P. (1995). High fertilization and pregnancy rate after intracytoplasmatic sperm injection with spermatozoa obtained from testicle biopsy. *Hum. Reprod.*, 10(1), 148

Related subjects: azoospermia, congenital absence vas deferens, diabetes mellitus, electro-ejaculation, micro-epididymal sperm aspiration, percutaneous epididymal sperm aspiration, spermatocele, spinal cord injury, testicular sperm aspiration, vibratory stimulation

SPERM FUNCTION TESTING

In contrast to the descriptive parameters of semen analysis with its low predictive value and mainly concentrating on numbers, the function of spermatozoa is more critical for the estimation of the fertility potential of a semen sample. Spermatozoa function defects can schematically be placed in the following categories (Table 43).

(1) Sperm–mucus interaction tests:

   (a) *in vivo*: postcoital tests; and

   (b) *in vitro*: slide test, sperm–cervical mucus contact test or capillary tube test.

In patients with negative postcoital tests, the abnormality may be due to the mucus (amount, antibodies, pH) or the spermatozoa (motility, antibodies). Spermatozoa and mucus can independently be assessed by crossed *in vitro* testing or the use of mucus substitutes such as bovine mucus. It must be realized that the penetration of antibody-coated spermatozoa is not retarded by these media.

(2) Acrosome reaction;

(3) Hypo-osmotic swelling test;

(4) Hemizona binding;

(5) Zona-free hamster egg penetration test;

(6) Reactive oxygen species generation; and

(7) Human *in vitro* fertilization test.

Table 43 The different types of sperm function testing

Defect	Tested by
Migration in female genital tract	progressive motility; sperm–mucus interaction tests; peritoneal sperm recovery; and hyperactivation
Binding to zona pellucida	acrosome reaction; hemizona binding; and human *in vitro* fertilization
Penetration of zona pellucida	electron microscopy after zona binding; hyperactivation; and human *in vitro* fertilization
Fusion with oolemma	zona-free hamster egg penetration; and human *in vitro* fertilization

The percentage of penetrated oocytes, or rather penetrated zonae, correlates best with fertilization *in vitro*. Therefore, the ultimate test for the infertile couple is the ability of the spermatozoa to fertilize the oocyte *in vitro*, although some doubt is justified as to whether the *in vitro* situation completely mimics the situation *in vivo*. As a result, a first *in vitro* fertilization cycle, regardless of the indication, bears a diagnostic character.

1. Aitken, R.J. (1995). Male infertility: prognostic value of old and new tests. *Assist. Reprod. Rev.*, 5(1), 26

2. Calvo, L., Dennison-Lagos, L., Banks, S.M. and Sherins, R.J. (1994). Characterization and frequency distribution of sperm acrosome reaction among normal and infertile men. *Hum. Reprod.*, 9(10), 1875

3. Cummins, J.M., Pember, S.M., Jequier, A.M., Yovich, J.L. and Hartmann, P.E. (1991). A test of the human sperm acrosome reaction following ionophore challenge: relationship to fertility and other seminal parameters. *J. Androl.*, 12, 98

4. Eggert-Kruse, W., Gerhard, I., Tilgen, W. and Runnebaum, B. (1989). Clinical significance of crossed *in vitro* sperm–cervical mucus penetration test in infertility inverstigation. *Fertil. Steril.*, 52, 1032

5. Hayes, M.F., Segal, S. and Moghissi, K.S. (1984). Comparison of the *in vitro* sperm penetration test using human cervical mucus and bovine estrus cervical mucus with the postcoital test. *Int. J. Fertil.*, 29, 133

6. Jeyendran, R.S., van der Ven, H.H. and Zaneveld, L.J. (1992). The hypo-osmotic swelling test: an update. *Arch. Androl.*, 29(2), 105

7. Liu, D.Y. and Baker, H.W.G. (1994). A new test for the assesment of sperm–zona pellucida penetration: relationship with results of other sperm tests and fertilization *in vitro*. *Hum. Reprod.*, 9(3), 489

8. Margalioth, E.J., Feinmesser, M., Navot, D., Mordel, N. and Bronson, R.A. (1989). The long-term predictive value of the zona-free hamster ova sperm penetration assay. *Fertil. Steril.*, 52, 490

9. Oehninger, S., Franken, D., Alexander, N. and Hodgen, G.D. (1992). Hemizona assay and its impact on the identification and treatment of human sperm. *Andrologia*, 24(6), 307

10. Sukcharoen, N., Keith, J., Irvine, D.S. and Aitken, R.J. (1995). Predicting the fertilization potential of human sperm suspensions *in vitro*: importance of sperm morphology and leukocyte contamination. *Fertil. Steril.*, 63(6), 1293

Related subjects: acrosome reaction — test, assisted reproduction, hemizona binding, hypo-osmotic swelling test, hyperactivation, in vitro fertilzation, motility, postcoital test, zona-free hamster egg penetration test

SPERMIATION

Release of the elongated spermatid from the Sertoli cell into the lumen of the seminiferous tubule, thus yielding the spermatozoon.

Related subjects: spermatogenesis

SPERMICIDES

Spermicides, which have been used for contraception since the 1950s, contain surface active agents damaging cell membranes including spermatozoa, bacteria and viruses. They are associated with reduction in risk of gonorrhea, pelvic inflammatory disease and *Chlamydia,* but not of *Trichomonas, Candida* or bacterial vaginosis. Most preparations contain nonoxynol-9, octoxynol-9 or menfegol. Epidemiological analysis, including recent meta-analysis, has shown insufficient evidence of a possible association between spermicide use and congenital abnormalities or possible abortions.

1. Barbone, F., Austin, H., Louv, W.C. and Alexander, W.J. (1990). A follow-up study of methods of contraception, sexual activity and rates of trichomoniasis, candidiasis and bacterial vaginosis. *Am. J. Obstet. Gynecol.*, 163, 510

2. Einarson, T.R., Koren, G., Mattice, D. and Schechter-Tsafriri, O. (1990). Maternal spermicide use and adverse reproductive outcome: a meta-analysis. *Am. J. Obstet. Gynecol.*, 162, 655

3. Niruthisard, S., Roddy, R.E. and Chutivongse, S. (1992). Use of nonoxynol-9 and reduction in rate of gonococcal and chlamydial cervical infection cervical infections. *Lancet*, 339, 1371

Related subjects: sexually transmitted diseases

SPERM MATURATION

Sperm maturation can be defined as the process starting with a spermatogonium undergoing mitosis as a first step in the spermatogenesis and the end stage being the fusion of the male and the female chromosomes establishing the genotype of a new individual. It is described in Table 44.

1. Acosta, A.A. (1994). Process of fertilization in the human and its abnormalities: diagnostic and therapeutic possibilities. *Obstet. Gynecol. Surv.*, 49(8), 567

Table 44 The process of sperm maturation

Maturation	Aim	Site	Testing
Intratesticular	complete spermato-genesis (70 days)	seminiferous tubules from basal layer towards lumen	chromosomal analysis testicular aspiration or biopsy hormonal evaluation
Extratesticular	acquire motility (14 days)	mainly in epididymis (head, body, tail) and ejaculatory ducts. Epididymal function largely depends on high local levels of testosterone and 5α-dihydrotestosterone	semen analysis
	acquire fertilization capacity	in part in the epididymis, also in the female genital tract (or *in vitro*); capacitation, hyper-activation, acrosomal reaction, penetration, fusion and decondensation	sperm function tests

Related subjects: acrosome reaction, capacitation, endocrinology, epididymis, hyperactivation, motility, semen analysis — normal values, spermatogenesis, testicular biopsy

SPERM PENETRATION ASSAY

Also known as zona-free hamster egg penetration test.

Related subjects: sperm function test, zona-free hamster egg penetration

SPERM PREPARATION TECHNIQUES (Table 45)

Spermatozoa lose their functional capacity rapidly during prolonged exposure to seminal plasma after ejaculation. Motility and viability decline markedly. Seminal plasma inhibits capacitation and the acrosome reaction and thus decreases the fertilizing capacity. Therefore, when semen has to be examined or to be used for clinical treatment, it has to be separated from the seminal plasma as soon as possible. To minimize the risk of infection, if semen is to be used for insemination thus bypassing the natural protection of the cervix, collection and handling have to be performed under optimal sterile conditions. For the same reason antibiotics, commonly in the form of penicillin plus streptomycin, are often added to the medium.

Table 45 The sperm preparation techniques

Techniques	Method	Comment
Dilution, washing, centrifugation		to be abandoned; all types of spermatozoa and other cells present in final selection; generation of reactive oxygen species by leukocytes and immature sperm cells
Migration (potentially functional spermatozoa migrate from liquefied semen into culture medium)	swim-up from semen	simple reliable
	swim-up from washed pellet	suspect: pelleting of unselected spermatozoa; low results in male factor *in vitro* fertilization
	swim-up from washed sperm	suspect: pelleting of unselected spermatozoa; low results in male factor *in vitro* fertilization
	Sperm-Select	swim-up method which uses highly purified hyaluronidase in the culture method; equivalent results to swim-up from semen
	swim-down	used for albumin-gradient, originally proposed for separation of Y-bearing sperm
Selective washing (based on continuous or discontinuous gradients where spermatozoa during centrifugation reach a position according to their own density)	Percoll	good yield of motile sperm except where there is poor motility. Concerns: remaining particles in prepared semen and endotoxins found in some batches
	Nycodenz	better yield in case of abnormal semen? Difficult in handling
Adherence (dead or abnormal sperm stick to glass)	glass wool glass beads Sephadex	damage to sperm plasma membrane beads in final preparation? possibly of value if centrifugation is not necessary

In most patients spermatozoa recovered after swim-up techniques as well as after Percoll gradient separation are reported to have higher numbers of sperm cells with normal morphology. Some publications also report better nuclear maturation after Percoll gradient separation. Other reports mention improvement in the hemizona binding only after sperm preparation with TEST yolk buffer and pentoxifylline compared to swim-up and Percoll.

1. Aitken, R.J. and Clarkson, J.S. (1988). Significance of reactive oxygen species and antioxidants in defining the efficacy of sperm preparation techniques. *J. Androl.*, 9, 367

2. Gellert-Mortimer, S.T., Clarke, G.N., Baker, H.W.G., Hyne, R.V. and Johnston, W.H.I. (1988). Evaluation of Nycodenz and Percoll density gradients for the selection of motile human spermatozoa. *Fertil. Steril.*, 49, 335

3. Mortimer, D. (1990). Semen analysis and sperm washing techniques. In Gagnon, C. (ed.) *Controls of Sperm Motility: Biological and Clinical Aspects.* (Boca Raton: CRC Press)

4. Mortimer, D. (1991). Sperm preparation techniques and iatrogenic failures of *in vitro* fertilization. *Hum. Reprod.*, 6, 173

5. Sjoblom, P. and Wikland, A. (1991). Follow-up study of sperm preparation for *in vitro* fertilization by swim-up in a solution of hyaluronate. *Hum. Reprod.*, 6, 722

6. Yogev, L., Homonnai, Z.T., Gamzu, R., Amit, A., Lessing, J.B., Paz, G. and Yavetz, H. (1995). The use of hemizona assay in the evaluation of the optimal sperm preparation technique. *Hum. Reprod.*, 10(4), 851

7. Zavos, P.M. (1991). A new simple method for preparing spermatozoa for insemination using the new SpermPrep TM filtration method. *J. Androl. Suppl.*, P-58 (abstract 133)

8. van der Zwalmen, P., Bertin-Segal, G., Geerts, L., Debauche, C. and Schoysman, R. (1991). Sperm morphology and *in vitro* fertilization pregnancy rate: comparison between Percoll gradient centrifugation and swim-up procedures. *Hum. Reprod.*, 6, 581

Related subjects: anti-oxidants, insemination, Nycodenz, Percoll, oxygen — reactive species, swim-up

SPERM TRANSPORT

At ejaculation, 40–400 million spermatozoa are deposited into the posterior fornix of the vagina. Within 2 minutes motile spermatozoa can be recovered from the preovulatory cervical mucus. It is unlikely that the remaining vaginal pool of spermatozoa plays a role as a reservoir for further migration into to cervix. Probably one of every 5000 spermatozoa deposited in the vagina will enter the cervical mucus. It is possible that the spermatozoa that can be found in the cervical crypts serve as a receptacle, but in humans this has not been proven. About 6–9 minutes after insemination spermatozoa have been demonstrated in the uterine cavity and the Fallopian tube. Probably spermatozoa with good motility are able to pass the uterotubal junction which, in this regard, serves as a selection barrier. Studies suggest that one in every million spermatozoa deposited in the vagina will reach the oviduct. Some of these spermatozoa are stored in the isthmus where they show reduced motility, which changes into rapid motility upon transfer into the ampulla (the site of fertilization) or a culture medium.

1. Mortimer, D. (1973). *Practical Laboratory Andrology*. (Oxford: Oxford University Press)

2. Settlage, D.S., Motoshima, M. and Treadway, D.R. (1973). Sperm transport from the external cervical os to the Fallopian tubes in women: a time and quantitation study. *Fertil. Steril.*, 24, 655

Related subjects: postcoital test

SPINAL CORD INJURY

Semen from males with chronic spinal cord injury is usually abnormal, due to, for example, low volume, variable count and very often poor motility. In addition, specific defects in sperm cell morphology, as judged by strict criteria are seen (e.g. higher percentage of small heads, vacuolated heads and tail defects). Increased scrotal temperature does not explain the poor semen quality. Other factors thought to contribute to poor semen quality are: stasis of prostatic fluid, recurrent urinary tract infection, abnormalities in the hypothalamic–pituitary–testicular axis, antisperm antibodies, long-term use of various medications and the type of bladder management. Commonly, vibro- or electro-ejaculation are required to obtain semen. Various stimuli such as bladder distension or electro-stimulation can trigger autonomic dysreflexia in men with injury above T5 level. Ultimately, this reaction can lead to severe hypertension to be antagonized by sympatholytic drugs. Although the fertility prognosis for patients with spinal cord injury has greatly improved with assisted reproduction, pregnancy rates are still below normal. The literature reports much better semen quality when semen is collected (and frozen) in the acute phase after the injury, starting within 2 weeks with frequent sampling until the quality starts to deteriorate.

1. Brackett, N.L., Lynne, C.M., Weizman, M.S., Bloch, W.E. and Abae, M. (1994). Endocrine profiles and semen quality of spinal cord injured men. *J. Urol.*, 151, 114

2. Brackett, N.L., Lynne, C.M., Weizman, M.S., Bloch, W.E. and Padron, O.F. (1994). Scrotal and oral temperatures are not related to semen quality or serum gonadotropin levels in spinal cord injured men. *J. Androl.*, 15, 614

3. Mallidis, C., Lim, T.C., Hill, S.T., Skinner, D.J., Brown, D.J., Johnston, W.I.J. and Baker, H.W.G. (1994). Collection of semen from men in acute phase of spinal cord injury. *Lancet*, 343, 1072

4. Sedor, J.F. and Hirsch, I.H. (1995). Evaluation of sperm morpholgy of electro-ejaculates of spinal cord injured men by strict criteria. *Fertil. Steril.*, 63(5), 1125

Related subjects: anejaculation, electro-ejaculation, hypogonadotropic hypogonadism, paraplegia, retrograde ejaculation, scrotal temperature, vibratory stimulation

SPLIT EJACULATE

There are indications, both diagnostic and therapeutic, when it is necessary to collect the ejaculate in different fractions. The first part contains the majority of the spermatozoa, mainly from the prostate. The latter part is mainly composed of sperm and secretions of the seminal vesicle. The split ejaculate technique prevents dilution of the prostatic spermatozoa and exposure to seminal 'contamination' and to epididymal antibodies.

Related subjects: ejaculate — composition, hyperspermia, prostate, seminal vesicle

STAINS

These are listed in Table 46.

Related subjects: acrosome reaction – test, flow cytometry, microscopy, morphology – abnormal and normal, necrozoospermia, semen analysis – processing of sample

Table 46 The different stains used in the assessment of male infertility

Name	Constituents	Use	Comment
Eosin, nigrosin	eosin, nigrosin (counterstain)	supravital	useful for rapid vitality scoring; needs to be performed independently from morphology testing
Triple stain	trypan blue, Bismarck brown, rose Bengal	supravital	reliability for acrosome reaction testing controversial because of instability of rose Bengal; length of procedure
Bryans	fast green, naphthol yellow S, methylene blue, pyronin Y	morphology acrosome	useful for morphology in post-Percoll specimens, where regular stains do not stain tail and membranes; AR use questionable; not good for fresh (i.e. light background)
Diff-Quick (commercial)	triarylmethane, thiazine, azure A, methylene blue, xanthene	morphology	commonly used in many centres; rapid and efficient stain
Giemsa	Giemsa	morphology	
Papanicolaou	hematoxylin orange G6, eosin Y, Bismarck brown, light green SF, morphology		
Shorr	hematoxylin, Shorr	morphology	
SperMac (commercial)		morphology acrosome	
TBP	toluidine blue, pyronine	morphology	
Testsimplets (commercial)	prestained slides, *n*-methylene blue, cresylviolet acetate		high background staining not in common use since Diff-Quick
Acridine orange	acridine orange	supravital	requires fluorescent microscope; now more commonly used in flow cytometry; slides are often cumbersome and demand lengthy procedure; results tend to subjection
Bis-benzimide		supravital	as before
FITC/TRITC	usually conjugated to lectins or antibodies	acrosome	as before
EB/PI	ethidium bromide/ propidium iodide	supravital	as before

AR = acrosome reaction, FITC = fluorescent iso-thiocyanide, TRITC = texas red iso-thiocyanide, EB/PI = ethidium bromide/propidium iodide

STATISTICS, FERTILITY

Statistical evaluation of fertility data is characterized by specific problems:

(1) Infertility is the result of a combination of contributions from two different individuals. The prognosis for couples with an abnormal male factor (at least one abnormal semen analysis according to World Health Organization criteria) is significantly affected by duration of infertility and history of previous pregnancy in the female partner, as shown by both univariate and multivariate analyses;

(2) For a valid evaluation, prediction or prognosis when counselling the patients, multiple variables have to be considered;

(3) Standardization of fertility variables is often lacking. Semen analysis, as an important indicator of male fertility potential, is a composed of several dissimilar parameters which do not necessarily reflect the same function or the fertilizing ability. There is no agreement in the literature regarding normality and hence predictive value of semen analysis;

(4) There is no consistent method for analyzing the results. Life-table analysis, for example, is a method which corrects for variation in duration of follow-up and losses to follow-up; and

(5) Finally, when evaluating statistical analyses applied to fertility data, it is important to be aware of the end-point parameters used. Preferably, pregnancy or live birth should be used as the end result of fertility studies that compare various methods.

Choosing a specific model for the interpretation of male infertility data may lead to a completely different results. Recently, a previous report about the assumed deterioration of male fertility which caused great amount of public interest was reassessed, employing alternative statistical approaches. These lead to different conclusions compared to the original publication. Perhaps the introduction of neural network computing into the evaluation of fertility data will enhance both prepredictibility and interpretation of infertility data because of its potential to take into account the above mentioned factors.

1. Bartoov, B., Eltes, F., Pansky, M., Lederman, H., Caspi, E. and Soffer, Y. (1993). Estimating fertility potential via semen analysis data. *Hum. Reprod.*, 8(1), 65

2. Cramer, D.W., Walker, A.M. and Schiff, I. (1979). Statistical methods in evaluating the outcome of infertility therapy. *Fertil. Steril.*, 32, 80

3. Duleba, A.J., Rowe, T.C., Ma, P. and Collins, J.A. (1992). Prognostic factors in assesment and management of male infertility. *Hum. Reprod.*, 7(10), 1388

4. Lamb, D.J. and Niederberger, C.S. (1993). Artificial intelligence in medicine and male infertility. *J. Urol.*, 11(2), 129

5. O'Donovan, P.A., Vandekerckhove, P., Lilford, R.J. and Hughes, E. (1993). Treatment of male infertility: is it effective? Review and meta-analyses of published randomized controlled trials. *Hum. Reprod.*, 8, 1209

6. Olsen, G.W., Bodner, K.M., Ramlow, J.M., Ross, C.E. and Lipshultz, L.I. (1995). Have sperm counts really been reduced in 50 years? A statistical model revisited. *Fertil. Steril.*, 63(4), 887

Related subjects: postcoital test, semen analysis — normal values — predictive value

STRESS

In stress activation, corticotropin releasing hormone and subsequently opioid mechanisms suppress gonadotropin releasing hormone activity, resulting in decreased pulsatile luteinizing hormone release. Prolactin levels are significantly higher in chronically stress-exposed men than in controls. The semen parameters show lower motility and increased abnormal morphology. Semen morphology seems to be particularly sensitive to stress.

1. Feichtinger, W. (1991). Environmental factors and fertility. *Hum. Reprod.*, 6(8), 1170

2. Gerhard, I., Lenhard, K., Eggert-Kruse, W. and Runnebaum, B. (1992). Clinical data which influence semen parameters in infertile men. *Hum. Reprod.*, 7, 830

3. Giblin, P., Poland, M., Moghissi, K., Ager, J. and Olson, J. (1988). Effects of stress and characteristic adaptability on semen quality in healthy men. *Fertil. Steril.*, 49, 127

Related subjects: history — male infertility, hypogonadotropic hypogonadism, hyperprolactinemia

STRICT CRITERIA

Morphology classified under strict criteria (Kruger's, Tygerberg, see Table 47) shows better predictive value for results of *in vitro* fertilization in comparison with the classical WHO criteria (see normal morphology). The criteria have changed over time since first published in 1986. Other authors have used the same terminology with different criteria.

Table 47 The strict criteria for the morphological classification of sperm

	Kruger et al. 1986	*Kruger et al. 1988*	*Menkveld et al. 1990*	*Kobayashi et al. 1991*
Length	no data	5–6 μm	3–5 μm	4–6 μm
Width	no data	2.5–3.5 μm	2–3 μm	2.4–3.5 μm
L/W ratio	no data	no data	1.5–1.67	no data
Stain	Papanicolaou	Diff-Quick	Papanicolaou	Diff-Quick
Cut-off	> 14% for normal fertilization rate in IVF	> 14% for normal fertilization rate in IVF, < 4% for very poor fertilization rate	no data	< 12% for lower pregnancy rate/IVF cycle

L/W ratio = length/width ratio, IVF = *in vitro* fertilization

1. Barratt, C.L.R. (1995). On the accuracy and clinical value of semen laboratory tests. *Hum. Reprod.*, 10(2), 247

2. Kobayashi, T., Jinno, M., Sugimura, K., Nozawa, S., Sugiyama, T. and Iida, E. (1991). Sperm-morphological assesment based on strict criteria and *in vitro* fertilization outcome. *Hum. Reprod.*, 6, 983

3. Kruger, T.F. and Menkveld, R., Stander, F.S.H., Lombard, C.J., van der Merwe, P.J., van Zy, J.A. and Smith, K. (1986). Sperm morphologic features as a prognostic factor in *in vitro* fertilization. *Fertil. Steril.*, 46, 1118

4. Kruger, T.F., Acosta, A.A., Simmons, K.F., Swanson, R.J., Matta, J.F. and Oehninger, S. (1988). Predictive value of abnormal sperm morphology (strict citeria) in *in vitro* fertilization. *Fertil. Steril.*, 49, 112

5. Menkveld, R., Stander, F.S.H., Kotze, T.J.W., Kruger, T.F. and van Zyl, J.A. (1990). The evaluation of morphological characteristics of human spermatozoa according to stricter criteria. *Hum. Reprod.*, 5, 586

Related subjects: *in vitro* fertilization, morphology — abnormal, morphology — normal, poor prognosis pattern morphology

SUBZONAL INSEMINATION (SUZI)

Usually around five spermaotzoa are injected into the perivitelline space of the oocyte. This limited number is chosen to limit the incidence of multiple sperm penetration into the oocyte. The method circumvents binding to and penetration through the zona pellucida. Some form of selection during membrane fusion is maintained, since the fusing spermatozoon has to be capacitated and acrosome reacted. The method has a reported fertilization percentage of at about 20.

1. Lippi, J., Mortimer, D. and Jansen, R.P.S. (1993). Subzonal insemination for extreme male factor infertility. *Hum. Reprod.*, 8, 908–15.

2. Ng, S., Bongso, A., Ratnam, S.S., Sathnanthan, H., Chan, C.L.K. and Wong, P.C. (1988). Pregnancy after transfer of sperm under zona. *Lancet*, ii, 790.

3. Palermo, G.D., Cohen, J., Alikani, M., Adler, A. and Rosenwaks, Z. (1995). Intracytoplasmic sperm injection: a novel treatment for all forms of male factor infertility. *Fertil. Steril.*, 63(6), 1231

Related subjects: micromanipulation

SWIM-UP

A sperm preparation technique which tries to separate functional spermatozoa through migration from liquefied, washed or pelleted semen into overlaying culture medium.

Related subjects: sperm preparation techniques

SYPHYLIS

The sexually transmitted disease caused by the spirochete *Treponema pallidum*. It cannot be cultured *in vitro*, but can be seen with dark-field microscopy. The diagnosis is based on non-specific test as VDRL, but have to be confirmed by a specific test, such as FTA-ABS, because of the high number of false-positive tests. The disease is characterized by three stages: primary (chancre), secondary after 1–3 months (systemic illness with rashes, fever and lymphadenopathy) and a late stage which may have a benign course, or show cardiac or neurological involvement. Epidemiologically, there is an increasing association with human autoimmune deficiency syndrome. Treatment consists of penicillin or doxycyclin.

1. Hutchinson, C.M. and Hook, E.W. III (1990). Syphilis in adults. *Med. Clin. N. Am.*, 74, 1389

2. Zenilman, J.M. (1992). Update on bacterial sexually transmitted disease. In Mellinger, B.C. and Smith, A.D. (eds.) Sexually transmitted diseases. *Urol. Clin. N. Am.*, 19(1) 25

Related subjects: acquired immunodeficiency syndrome, sexually transmitted diseases

T*t*

TAIL DEFECTS

Tail defects, such as those shown in Figure 31, impair sperm motility. There is a spectrum of abnormalities varying from ultrastructural (immotile-cilia syndrome including Kartagener's syndrome, Young's syndrome, drug addiction) to gross defects. Functional abnormalities associated with a normal axonema also are seen. No specific therapy is available to normalize the motility. Therefore *in vitro* fertilization and micromanipulation is currently the treatment of choice.

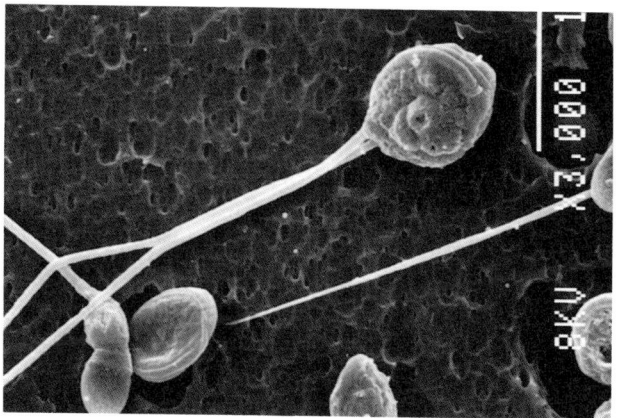

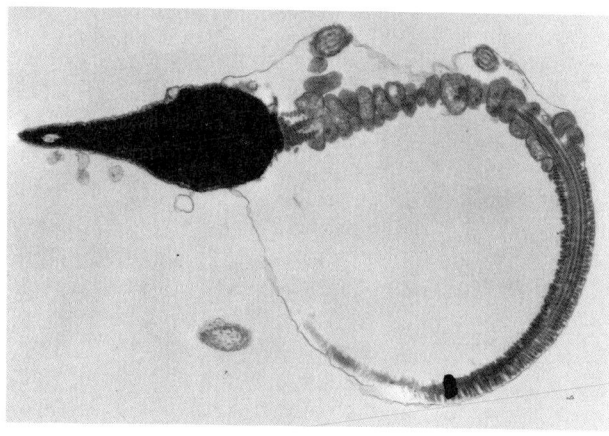

Figure 31 Some examples of tail defects: (A) a scanning electron micrograph showing a double tail; and (B) a transmission electron micrograph of a Dag defect (coiled tail)

Related subjects: asthenozoospermia, immotile cilia syndrome, Kartagener's syndrome, microscopy, morphology — abnormal, Young's syndrome

TAMOXIFEN

This is an anti-estrogen that exhibits less estrogenic activity than clomiphene citrate. The usual dose is 20–30 mg/day for 3–6 months. As with clomiphene citrate, its positive effect on semen parameters is not proven in randomized controlled studies.

1. Krause, W., Holland-Moritz, H. and Schramm, P. (1992). Treatment of idiopathic oligozoospermia with tamoxifen. A randomized controlled study. *Int. J. Androl.*, 15, 14

2. O'Donovan, P., Vandekerchhove, P., Lilford, R. and Hughes, E. (1993). Treatment of male infertility. Is it effective? Review and meta analysis of published randomized controlled trials. *Hum. Reprod.*, 8, 1209

3. Sterzik, K., Rosenbusch, B. and Magck, J. (1993). Tamoxifen treatment of oligozoospermia. Re-evaluation of its effects including additional sperm function tests. *Arch. Gynecol. Obstet.*, 252, 143

Related subjects: clomiphene citrate, medication — treatment

TAURINE

Hypotaurine and taurine are both substances essentially derived from cysteine. They are secreted in human oviduct epithelial cells, are also found in follicular fluid and can be detected in seminal fluid and spermatozoa. Due to their antioxidant properties they play an important role in the protection of spermatozoa against peroxidative damage. *In vitro*, the compounds are reported to be necessary for capacitation, fertilization and early embryonic development.

1. Guerin, P., Guillaud, J. and Menezo, Y. (1995). Hypotaurine in spermatozoa and genital secretions and its production by oviduct epithelial cells *in vitro*. *Hum. Reprod.*, 10(4), 866

Related subjects: anti-oxidants, hypotaurine, oxygen — reactive species, sperm preparation

TERATOZOOSPERMIA

Teratozoospermia is abnormal sperm morphology. Sperm defects can affect the sperm head (tapering, vacuolated), midpiece (thin midpiece), and tail (hairpin, coiled), but most coexist in the same specimen. If the percentage of abnormal spermatozoa in a semen specimen exceeds a certain limit, the fecundity rate decreases. This threshold value is preferably defined in each laboratory. However, standard percentages of normal sperm are set by World Health Organisation (50%), or by several authors, such as Kruger (14%), each using different criteria for normality. A single homogeneous morphological abnormality is the least common sperm abnormality (1%), e.g. acrosomal agenesis (round-head or globospermia).

Related subjects: morphology — abnormal, strict criteria

TESTICULAR ATROPHY

The testes are small and soft. Clinical features include azoospermia or severe oligospermia in the face of elevated gonadotropins. Histologically, there is peritubular fibrosis, interstitial fibrosis and tubular sclerosis. It is an end stage of a disease process affecting the testis. It has to be mentioned that histology obtained from needle aspiration or testicular biopsy is not necessarily completely representative for the entire testis and, therefore, does not exclude the presence of some remaining spermatogenesis beyond the spermatid stage. Presently, only few spermatozoa (obtained from testicular biopsy) seem to be necessary to proceed to fertilization and pregnancy if intracytoplasmic sperm injection and *in vitro* fertilization are applied.

1. Yemini, M., Vanderzwalmen, P., Mukaida, T., Schoengold, S. and Birkenfeld, A. (1995). Intracytoplasmic sperm injection, fertilization and embryo transfer after retrieval of spermatozoa by testicular biopsy from an azoospermic male with testicular tubular atrophy. *Fertil. Steril.*, 63(5), 1118

Related subjects: acquired immunodeficiency syndrome, azoospermia, hypergonadotropic hypogonadism, intracytoplasmic sperm injection, liver disease, mumps, testicular biopsy — histopathology

TESTICULAR BIOPSY

Testicular biopsy is indicated in patients with azoospermia, normal testis and normal or slightly elevated gonadotropins. The aim is to differentiate between ductal obstruction (vas deferens, epididymis) and germ cell pathology. Severe oligozoospermia (less than 5 million/ml) is also an indication for testicular biopsy in order to rule out partial obstruction (epididymis, vas deferens, ejaculatory ducts). The procedure is best performed either under general or regional (spinal/epidural) anesthesia. If local anesthesia is used, a blind procedure for this should be avoided in order to prevent injury to the spermatic cord. The biopsy should be bilateral, since differences do occur. Complications of the procedure include: inadvertent biopsying of the epididymis with subsequent obstruction, hematoma and infection.

Before performing testicular biopsy, consider whether the procedure should be combined with testicular sperm aspiration for direct use or cryopreservation.

1. Magid, M.S., Cash, K.L. and Goldstein, M. (1990). The testicular biopsy in the evaluation of infertility. *Semin. Urol.*, 8, 51

2. Goldstein, M. (1992). Surgery of male infertility and other scrotal disorders. In Walsh,

P.C., Retik, A.B., Stamey, T.A. and Vaughan, E.D. (eds.) *Campbell's Urology*, 6th edn. (Philadelphia: W.B. Saunders)

Related subjects: azoospermia, cryopreservation, intracytoplasmic sperm injection, testicular sperm aspiration

TESTICULAR BIOPSY, HISTOPATHOLOGY OF (Table 48)

Table 48 The frequency of different conditions observed in the histopathology of a testicular biopsy

Diagnosis	Comment	Frequency range as observed in testicular biopsy specimen (%)
Normal spermatogenesis	in combination with azoo- or oligozoospermia: obstruction or suspected partial obstruction	3–20
Hypospermatogenesis	all stages of spermatogenesis present but proportionate reduction at each level; may be caused by any factor interfering with hypo-thalamic–pituitary–testicular axis	9–51
Maturation arrest	failure to progress; usually at primary spermatocyte level; can be complete or incomplete, in the latter case dysproportional reduction is seen	1–32
Sertoli cell-only syndrome	germ cell aplasia; complete or incomplete form; often idiopathic, can be seen after infection, radio-therapy or chemotherapy	8–16
Sclerosing tubular generation	characteristic for Klinefelter's syndrome	3–9
(Peri)tubular fibrosis	end-stage of testicular damage with loss of germ cells, loss of Sertoli cells and atrophy of Leydig cells; reported after ischemia, mumps, iradiation, cryptorchidism, etc.	1–6

1. Magid, M.S., Cash, K.L. and Goldstein, M. (1990). The testicular biopsy in the evaluation of infertility. *Semin. Urol.*, 8, 51

2. Wheeler, J.E. (1991). Histology of the fertile and infertile testis. In Kraus, F.T., Damjanov, I. and Kaufman, N. (eds.) *Pathology of Reproductive Failure*. (Baltimore: Williams and Wilkins)

Related subjects: fine needle aspiration, Klinefelter's syndrome, Sertoli cell-only syndrome, spermatogenic arrest, testicular atrophy

TESTICULAR CANCER

Testicular cancer is the most common malignancy of men between the age of 20 and 40 years. The incidence of testicular cancer has increased two- to four-fold over the last 50 years. This increase, like the increase in maldescent of testis and hypospadia, may be related to environmental factors, since all could be reflections of errors in normal development during fetal life. Because similar abnormalities are found in males exposed to stilbestrol during fetal life, this increase might be related to increased estrogen exposure *in utero*. Sources for these estrogens are possibly: recycling of synthetic estrogens (human, livestock), consumption of cow's milk, phyto-estrogens and so-called estrogenic (often organochloric) chemicals. In up to 60% of men with unilateral testicular cancer, severely impaired spermatogenesis is reported to be found before radiation and/or chemotherapeutics, as shown by testicular biopsy (25% irreversible spermatogenic arrest), semen analysis and hormonal parameters. Fertility-related problems after treatment include postsurgical sequela such as antisperm antibodies, anejaculation or retrograde ejaculation. In addition, the application of radiation and cytostatic therapy can deteriorate semen quality. Several animal studies have suggested that protection of rapidly dividing spermatogonia against the damage of chemotherapy can be achieved by pretreatment suppression with androgens or gonadotropin-releasing hormone agonists, but data in humans so far have been inconclusive. Cryopreservation of spermatozoa, even of poor quality, should always be included in the treatment plan, since the introduction of modern assisted reproductive techniques, especially micromanipulation, has greatly improved the future fertility prospect for these patients.

1. Berthelsen, J.G. and Skakkebaek, N.S. (1983). Gonadal fuction in men with testis cancer. *Fertil. Steril.*, 39(1), 68

2. Presti, J.C., Herr, H.W. and Carroll, P.R. (1993). Fertility and testis cancer. In Klein, E.A. and Kay, R. (eds.) Testis cancer in adults and children. *Urol. Clin. N. Am.*, 20(1), 173

3. Sharpe, R.M. and Skakkebaek, N.S. (1994). Are oestrogens involved in falling sperm counts and disorders of the male reproductive tract? *Lancet*, 341, 1392

Related subjects: anejaculation, chemotherapy, cryopreservation, cryptorchidism, radiation, retrograde ejaculation, spermatogenic arrest

TESTICULAR EXPLORATION AND SPERM EXTRACTION (TESE)

A method in which the testis is carefully examined for the presence of sperm cells. If found, the sperm cells are used for intracytoplasmic sperm injection. The indication for the technique is in males with infertility signified by

165

azoospermia, high gonadotropins and histopathology reports like Sertoli cell-only, spermatogenic arrest or testicular atrophy.

1. Silber, S.J., van Steirteghem, A.C. and Devroey, P. (1995). Sertoli cell revisited. *Hum. Reprod.*, 10(5), 1031

Related subjects: Sertoli cell-only, testicular atrophy, testicular biopsy — histopathology

TESTICULAR FAILURE

This is a general description meaning that the testis, even after treatment, fails to produce spermatozoa. Presently only few conditions ultimately exhibit 'failure' since, as discussed elsewhere, very often even in cases of so-called atrophy, it is possible to obtain spermatozoa by means of aspiration or biopsy. These spermatozoa then are successfully utilized for intracytoplasmic sperm injection in combination with *in vitro* fertilization.

Related subjects: hypergonadotropic hypogonadism, Sertoli-cell only syndrome, testicular atrophy, testicular biopsy — histopathology

TESTICULAR FEMINIZATION SYNDROME

A term used for individuals who are genotypically male (46XY) and phenotypically female. The underlying disorder is androgen receptor abnormality and therefore part of the androgen resistance or insensitivity syndrome. Patients with the testicular feminization syndrome represent one end of the spectrum, exhibiting the classical and complete form of androgen resistance. They have functional testes which can be located in the inguinal region, sometimes in a hernia. These individuals lack facial, axillary and pubic hair. They have female external genitalia and a normally developed distal two-thirds of the vagina. The proximal third of the vagina, the uterus and the Fallopian tubes are absent due to production of anti-Mullerian hormone produced by functional Sertoli cells at the time of testicular differentiation. Testosterone, estradiol and luteinizing hormone levels are high, whereas follicle stimulating hormone is normal. Testicular biopsy shows immature germ cells and hyperplastic Leydig cells.

1. Griffin, J.E. (1992). Androgen resistance — the clinical and molecular spectrum. *N. Engl. J. Med.*, 326, 611

Related subjects: androgen insensitivity syndrome

TESTICULAR SPERM ASPIRATION (TESA)

Spermatozoa can be obtained from testicular biopsies and be used for *in vitro* fertilization in combination with a micromanipulation procedure. Although the maturation process in the epididymis is bypassed, fertilization and pregnancy rates are reported to be comparable to spermatozoa retrieved from the epididymis.

1. Schoysman, R., Vanderzwalmen, P., Nijs, M., Segal, L., Segal-Bertin, G., Geerts, L., van Roosendaal, E. and Schoysman-Deboeck, A. (1993). Pregnancy after fertilization with human testicular spermatozoa. *Lancet*, 342, 1236

2. Silber, S.J., van Steirteghem, A.C., Liu, J., Nagy, Z., Tournaye, H. and Devroey, P. (1995). High fertilization and pregnancy rate after intracytoplasmic sperm injection with spermatozoa obtained from testicle biopsy. *Hum. Reprod.*, 10(1), 148

Related subjects: azoospermia, intracytoplasmic sperm injection, testicular biopsy

TESTIS

Functionally the testis can be distinguished to consist of two main parts:

(1) The interstitial tissue containing Leydig cells, stroma and blood and lymph vessels. The main function is endocrine, signified by the production of testosterone and estradiol.

(2) The seminiferous tubules with spermatogonia and Sertoli cells. These cells are separated by the blood–testis barrier, dividing it in two compartments: the basal and the adluminal. Its foremost function is exocrine: spermatogenesis. The Sertoli cells secrete inhibin. The average testicular size is 5.0×3.0 cm and the volume at adult age is 24 ± 4 ml, decreasing in elderly men. Of the total volume, about 80% consists of seminiferous tubules, so that estimation of the testicular volume gives a rough estimate of spermatogenic cell capacity.

1. Mortimer, D. (1994). *Practical Laboratory Andrology*. (Oxford: Oxford University Press)

Related subjects: anatomy, endocrinology, physical examination — male infertility, Leydig cell, Sertoli cell

TESTIS DETERMINING FACTOR (TDF)

This factor is necessary for differentiation of the bipotential gonad into a testis. It is located in region 1 of the short arm of the Y chromosome (Yp1). TDF is found in the same region as the sex determining region (SRY) and these genes are probably identical. In some patients with intact SRY and 46XY genotype, complete lack of testicular differentiation has been found, suggesting that other factors besides SRY are needed for complete gonadal determination.

1. Behzaian, M., Tho, S.P.T. and McDonough, P.G. (1991). SGI transactions: the presence of the testicular determining sequence, SRY, in 46XY females with gonadal dysgenesis (Swyer syndrome). *Am. J. Obstet. Gynecol.*, 165, 1887

2. Berta, P., Hawkins, J.R. and Sinclair, A.H. (1990). Genetic evidence equating SRY and the testis-determining factor. *Nature*, 348, 448

3. Mittwoch, U. (1993). Identical SRY mutations with different phenotypic effects. *Am. J. Hum. Genet.*, 1272

Related subjects: testis determining factor, Y chromosome

TESTOSTERONE

Testosterone is a steroid hormone mainly produced by the Leydig cells. Biosynthesis and secretion are primarily dependent on luteinizing hormone secretion. Testosterone has a negative feedback on luteinizing hormone secretion through action on hypothalamic and pituitary level. About 1–2% of the circulating testosterone is free in healthy men, 30% is bound to testosterone–estradiol binding globulin with high affinity and the remainder is much more weakly bound to albumin and other proteins. Testosterone action in target tissues can be exerted before or after conversion to dihydrotestosterone, after aromatization to estradiol or independent from androgen or estrogen receptors. It maintains spermatogenesis and serves as a prehormone for dihydrotestosterone and estradiol.

1. Veldhuis, J. (1991). The hypothalamic–pituitary–testicular axis. In Yen, S.S.C. and Jaffe, R.B. (eds.) *Reproductive Endocrinology*, 3rd edn. (Philadelphia: W.B. Saunders)

Related subjects: endocrinology, Leydig cell, testosterone–estradiol binding globulin

TESTOSTERONE–ESTRADIOL BINDING GLOBULIN (TEBG)

A β-globulin (also called sex hormone binding globulin, SHBG) that is the major carrier protein both for testosterone and estradiol. There is a close resemblance to androgen binding protein (ABP) produced by the Sertoli cells. Although about 1–2% of the circulating testosterone is free in healthy men, 30% is bound to TEBG with high affinity (the remainder is much more weakly bound to albumin and other proteins).

1. Veldhuis, J. (1991). The hypothalamic–pituitary–testicular axis. In Yen, S.S.C. and Jaffe, R.B. (eds.) *Reproductive Endocrinology*, 3rd edn. (Philadelphia: W.B. Saunders)

Related subjects: endocrinology, testosterone

TESTOSTERONE REBOUND THERAPY

Administration of testosterone derivatives has been reported to improve sperm count after a period of azoospermia produced by their inhibitory effects on gonadotropins. However, controlled studies did not show beneficial effects of testosterone rebound therapy. A number of patients treated with high-dose androgens had persistently decreased sperm density secondary to the treatment and even cases of permanent azoospermia have been reported.

1. Wang, C., Chan, C. and Wong, K. (1983). Comparison of the effectiveness of placebo clomiphene citrate, mesterolone, pentoxifylline and testosterone rebound therapy for the treatment of idiopathic oligospermia. *Fertil. Steril.*, 40, 358

Related subjects: androgen therapy, endocrinology, medication – treatment

TEST YOLK BUFFER

TEST (TES and Tris) yolk buffer (TYB) is used to enhance motility and for cryopreservation of sperm and then supplemented with 8% glycerol. Some reports sugggest that test yolk buffer enhances sperm fertilizing capacity in *in vitro* fertilization. Perhaps this is due to the fact that incubation of medium with TYB increases the occurrence of acrosome reaction and the penetration rates of the sperm penetration assay.

1. Jacobs, B.R., Caulfield, J. and Boldt, J. (1995). Analysis of TEST (TES and Tris) yolk buffer effects on human sperm. *Fertil. Steril.*, 63(5), 1064

2. Veeck, L.L. (1992). TES and Tris (TEST)-yolk buffer systems, sperm function testing, and *in vitro* fertilization. *Fertil. Steril.*, 58(3), 484

Related subjects: cryopreservation, culture media

THALASSEMIA

A congenital partly autosomal dominant blood disorder characterized by abnormal globin (HbC), hemolysis, anemia and defective erythropoiesis. Male infertility may be detected secondary to iron deposition in pituitary and testes. In case of pituitary failure, treatment with gonadotropins can be successful.

1. DeSanctis, V., Vullo, C. and Katz, M. (1988). Induction of spermatogenesis in thalassemia. *Fertil. Steril.*, 50, 969

Related subjects: hypogonadotropic hypogonadism

TORSION, TESTICULAR

Occurs mainly during adolescence, with a yearly incidence of 1/4000. Clinical symptoms develop in torsions of at least 360°. The greatest damage occurs after the first 8 hours. If the affected testis is left *in situ* for longer time, this will have a deleterious effect on the contralateral testes, probably on an immunological basis. Although early detorsion and orchidopexy or removal of the affected testicle is recommended, there is controversy as to whether this will preserve future fertility, since there are data suggesting that abnormal testicles are more likely to undergo torsion than normal testes.

1. Hagen, P., Buchholz, M.M. and Eigenmann, J. (1992). Testicular dysplasia causing disturbance of spermatogenesis in patients with unilateral torsion of the testis. *Urol. Int.*, 49, 154

2. Thomas, W.E.G., Cooper, M.J. and Crane, G.A. (1984). Testicular exocrine malfunction after torsion. *Lancet*, ii, 1357

Related subjects: spermatogenic arrest, ultrasound

TRANSFORMING GROWTH FACTOR (TGF)

The transforming growth factors are a group of proteins exerting different actions. They are involved in the local control of spermatogenesis affecting cell proliferation and meiosis in a paracrine and autocrine way. Recently transforming growth factor β, produced in the Sertoli cells, was demonstrated in the seminal plasma in an inactive form. TGF-β is known to have immunosuppressive activity. Activation of TGF-β takes place at a pH lower than 4, which corresponds to the natural acid environment in the vagina. TGF-β is therefore thought to exert immunoprotective activity for haploid sperm cells in the Sertoli cells and also in the vagina.

1. Nocera, M. and Ming Chu, T. (1995). Characterization of latent transforming growth factor from human seminal plasma. *Am. J. Reprod. Immunol.*, **33**, 282

Related subjects: spermatogenesis

TRICHOMONAS

Distal urethritis caused by *Trichomonas* is rare: it contributes 1% to non-gonococcal urethritis. The condition is diagnosed by identifying the parasite in a wet mount. There is no significant effect on male fertility.

1. Moskowitz, M.O. and Mellinger, B.C. (1992). Sexually transmitted diseases and their relation to male infertility. In Mellinger, B.C. and Smith, A.D. (eds.) *Urol. Clin. N. Am.*, **19**(1), 35

Related subjects: sexually transmitted diseases

TUBERCULOSIS

Tuberculous infection of testis, epididymis, seminal vesicles, prostate and penis can be blood-borne, sexually transmitted or occur as a complication of renal tuberculosis. The most frequent primary location of genitourinary tuberculosis is the epididymis. With prolonged infection fibrosis and obstruction do occur, primarily of the epididymis.

1. Gow, J.G. (1992). Genitourinary tuberculosis. In Walsh, P.C., Retik, A.B., Stamey, T.A. and Vaughan, E.D. (eds.) *Campbell's Urology*, 6th edn. (Philadelphia: W.B.Saunders)

Related subjects: epididymitis, hypogonadotropic hypogonadism

TYGERBERG CRITERIA

Alternative name for strict or Kruger's criteria after the hospital where the study was performed.

1. Kruger, T.F., Menkveld, R., Stander, F.S.H., Lombard, C.J., van der Merwe, P.J., van Zyl, J.A. and Smith, K. (1986). Sperm morphologic features as a prognostic factor in *in vitro* fertilization. *Fertil. Steril.*, **46**, 1118

Related subjects: strict criteria for sperm morphology

U u

ULTRASONOGRAPHY

Scrotal ultrasound

The normal adult testis is homogeneous on ultrasound and measures on average $4 \times 2.5 \times 2.5$ cm, which corresponds to a volume of 15–20 cc. The following abnormalities can be identified: solid tumors, torsion (no flow with color flow Doppler), epididymo-orchitis (increased flow CFD), abnormal size because of atrophy due to a varicocele, hydrocele and cysts. Varicocele itself can be seen with color flow Doppler, showing excellent correlation with venography.

Transrectal ultrasound (TRUS)

Seminal vesicles and vasal ampulla can be easily identified by transrectal ultrasonography, whereas the ejaculatory duct only is visible when obstructed. Indications for transrectal ultrasonography in male infertility are:

(1) Low-volume (< 1.5 ml) azoo- or oligozoospermia (< 5 million) in the presence of normal or slightly decreased size of the testes;

(2) Congenital absence of vas deferens;

(3) Retrograde ejaculation; and

(4) Hematospermia.

Transrectal ultrasonography has replaced vasography as the first-line diagnostic modality, especially for evaluation of ejaculatory duct obstruction.

1. Honig, S.C. (1994). New diagnostic techniques in the evaluation of anatomic abnormalities of the infertile male. *Urol. Clin. N. Am.*, 21(3), 418

Related subjects: azoospermia, congenital absence vas deferens, ejaculatory duct obstruction, hydrocele, magnetic resonance imaging, oligozoospermia/low volume flowsheet, torsion, varicocele, vasography, venography

UREAPLASMA UREALYTICUM

This organism is responsible for 25% of non-gonococcal urethritis. The diagnosis is made by exclusion. Doxycycline or quinolones are used as the therapy of choice. Therapy improves motility if it was decreased, but has no effect on conception rates.

1. Moskowitz, M.O. and Mellinger, B.C. (1992). Sexually transmitted diseases and their relation to male infertility. In Melinger, B.C. and Smith, A.D. (eds.) Sexually transmitted diseases. *Urol. Clin. N. Am.*, 19(1), 35

Related subjects: sexually transmitted diseases

V v

VARICOCELE

Varicocele is distension of the pampiniform plexus in the scrotum secondary to an increase in venous pressure. It is found in 15% of the general male population, in 35% of men with primary infertility and in 81% of men with secondary infertility. It is associated with a duration dependent reduction of testicular size and abnormalities in spermatogenesis. Grading is from mild (grade I, only palpated by Valsalva's maneuver), to moderate (grade II, easily palpated) and large (grade III, visible bulging of scrotal skin). Varicocelectomy can be performed in several ways: retroperitoneal, inguinal (conventional or microsurgical), laparoscopic or radiographic occlusion with balloon or coil. Complications of the procedure include the formation of a hydrocele, injury to the testicular artery and recurrence of the varicocele. Varicocelectomy has been shown to improve testicular volume and sperm count. It may be that early repair of varicocele at adolescent age, especially in men with abnormal semen analysis and decreased testicular volume of the affected side eventually will prove to be of value. However, the positive effect of varicocelectomy as measured by pregnancy rates has yet to be demontrated by randomized studies. The only prospective, randomized controlled studies so far were performed in an adolescent population and addressed sperm count but not infertility.

1. Goldstein, M. (1995). Varicocelectomy: general considerations – complications and results. In Goldstein, M. (ed.) *Surgery for Male Infertility.* (Philadelphia: W. B. Saunders)

2. Hargreave, T.B. (1993). Varicocele – a clinical enigma. *Br. J. Urol.,* 72(4), 401

3. Kass, E.J. and Reitelman, C. (1995). Adolescent varicocele. In Kaplan, G.W. (ed.) Common problems in pediatric urology. *Urol. Clin. N. Am.,* 22(1), 151

4. Laven, J.S.E., Haans, L.C.F. and Mali, W.P.T.M. (1992). Effects of varicocele treatment in adolescents: a randomized study. *Fertil. Steril.,* 58, 756

5. Okuyama, A., Nakamura, M. and Namiki, M. (1988). Surgical repair of varicocele at puberty: preventive treatment for fertility improvement. *J. Urol.,* 139, 562

Related subjects: asthenozoospermia, leukocytospermia, physical examination — male infertility, scrotal temperature, spermatogenic arrest, ultrasonography, venography

VASECTOMY, REVERSAL

After successful reversal of vasectomy sperm count slowly recovers, to reach a plateau after 6 months. Patency rates depend on the technique (macroscopically or microscopically) and the experience of the surgeon. There is a direct relationship between the time since vasectomy and pregnancy rate:

(1) < 3 years: 75%.

(2) 3–8 years: 50%.

(3) 9–14 years: 40%.

(4) > 15 years: 30%.

Literature reports 44–81% pregnancy rates after reversal of vasectomy. Failure may be caused by:

(1) Stenosis or blockage of the vaso-vasostomy.

(2) Epididymal blockage. Back pressure from the vasectomy site may lead to rupture of epididymal tubules and local sperm granulosa formation.

(3) Antibody formation response to vasectomy. In 60-80% of vasectomized men sperm antibodies can be found. Especially high titers of IgA are associated with infertility.

(4) Spermatogenesis has ceased. Although very uncommon it should always be considered.

1. Belker, A.M., Thomas, A.J. Jr, Fuchs, E.F., Konnak, J.W. and Sharlip, I.D. (1991). Results of 1469 microsurgical vasectomy reversals by the vasovasostomy study group. *J. Urol.*, 141, 505

2. Hendry, W.F. (1994). Vasectomy and vasectomy reversal. *Br. J. Urol.*, 73, 337

Related subjects: antisperm antibodies, vasovasostomy

VASOEPIDIDYMOSTOMY

Causes for epididymal obstruction can be brought into the following catagories:

(1) Congenital: absence of distal part together with absent vas, Young's syndrome.

(2) Infection: history of epididymitis (tuberculosis, *Chlamydia*).

(3) Trauma: injury or during surgery (testicular biopsy, hydrocele).

(4) After vasectomy.

In case of epididymal obstruction, several microsurgical reanastamosis procedures (end-to-end and end-to-side) between vas deferens and epididymis have been described. Patency rates of 39–85% and pregnancy rates from 13 to 42% have been reported. In case of partial obstruction, microsurgical correction versus epididymal or testicular sperm aspiration in combination with intracytoplasmic sperm injection have to be considered.

1. Dewire, D.M. and Thomas, A.J. (1995). Indications for vasoepididymostomy. In Goldstein, M. (ed.) *Surgery of Male Infertility*. (Philadelphia: W. B. Saunders)

2. Hauser, R., Temple-Smith, P.D., Southwick, G.J., McFarlane, J. and de Kretser, D.M. (1995). Pregnancies after microsurgical correction of partial epididymal and vasal obstruction. *Hum. Reprod.*, 10(5), 1152

3. Thomas, A.J. and Howards, S.S. (1991). Microsurgical treatment of male infertility. In Lipshultz, L.I. and Howards, S.S. (eds.) *Infertility in the Male*, p. 357. (St Louis: Mosby Year Book)

Related subjects: congenital absence of vas deferens, history in male infertility, microsurgery, vasectomy reversal, Young's syndrome

VASOGRAPHY

Vasography is still to be considered the gold standard for identification of distal ejaculatory duct obstruction and obstruction of the vas deferens proximal to the vasal ampulla. It is indicated when inguinal vasal obstruction is suspected in order to determine the site of obstruction and also in cases of low volume azoo- or oligozoospermia with inconclusive transrectal ultrasonography. If testicular biopsy has shown spermatogenesis, vasography is usually performed during a scrotal exploration and possible microsurgical reconstruction. It can be performed employing different techniques: via vasopuncture, vasotomy, retrograde catheterization via cystoscopy or via transrectal puncture. A mixture of renografin and colored dye is injected distally.

1. Honig, S.C. (1994). New diagnostic techniques in the evaluation of anatomic abnormalities of the infertile male. *Urol. Clin. N. Am.*, 21(3), 425

Related subjects: azoospermia, ejaculatory duct obstruction, ultrasonography

VASOVASOSTOMY

Microsurgical reanastamosis of the vas deferens is mainly performed for reversal of vasectomy, and less commonly, in cases of vas deferens obstruction due to other causes. Patency rates of 90% and pregnancy of at about 50% are reported.

1. Belker, A.M., Thomas, A.J. Jr, Fuchs, E.F., Konnak, J.W. and Sharlip, I.D. (1991). Results of 1469 microsurgical vasectomy reversals by the vasovasostomy study group. *J. Urol.*, 141, 505

Related subjects: vasectomy — reversal

VENOGRAPHY

Retrograde spermatic venography is used for the diagnosis of varicocele. It has high sensitivity but, unfortunately, a low specificity (high false-positive results).

Related subjects: varicocele, ultrasonography

VIBRATORY STIMULATION, PENILE

In patients with disorders of ejaculation a vibrator is applied to the ventral surface of the penis close to the frenulum. Stimulation is usually performed for 5–20 minutes, or until ejaculation occurs. It seems essential that an adequate peak-to-peak amplitude is applied to exceed the ejaculatory threshold. In 60–80% of selected patients semen can be obtained this way, but if the method fails, electro-ejaculation has to be considered. No absolute predictors of ejaculatory success are available. Therefore, most patients with anejaculation and spinal cord lesions should be considered as candidates for vibratory stimalution.

1. Beckerman, H., Becher, J. and Lankhorst, G.J. (1993). The effectiviness of vibratory stimulation in anejaculatory men with spinal cord injury. *Paraplegia*, 31(11), 689

2. Sonksen, S.J., Biering-Sorensen, F. and Kristensen, J.K. (1994). Ejaculation induced by penile vibratory stimulation in men with spinal cord injuries. The importance of the vibratory amplitude. *Paraplegia*, 32(10), 651

Related subjects: anejaculation, electro-ejaculation, paraplegia, sperm collection techniques, spinal cord injury

X*x*

XYY MALE

The incidence is 1–4 per 1000 newborn males. Semen analysis ranges from normal values to azoospermia. The majority of affected individuals are fertile. Tall but otherwise normal phenotype is the rule. The majority of the affected men have normal levels of luteinizing hormone and follicle stimulating hormone, while a minority show elevated titers. Antisocial and aggressive behavior is reported in 1-2%, probably related to the diminished intellectual function.

1. Griffin, J.E. and Wilson, J.D. (1992). Disorders of sexual differentiation. In Walsh, P.C., Retik, A.B., Stamey, T.A. and Vaughan, A.D. (eds.) *Campbell's Urology*, Vol. 2. (Philadelphia: WB Saunders)

Related subjects: chromosomal abnormalities — somatic cells, hypergonadotropic hypogonadism, spermatogenic arrest

Y*y*

Y CHROMOSOME

The Y chromosome is a small acrocentric chromosome, with a short arm Yp and a long arm Yq. A heterochromatic part (distal Yq) genetically inactive and a euchromatic part can be distinguished: part of the latter is homologues with sequences on the X chromosome. On the short arm close to the pseudoautosomal region the testis determining factor (TDF) is located within the SRY (sex-related Y gene) region; they are probably identical. The azoospermia factor gene in control of spermatogenesis is located on the distal part of the long arm interval 6. Close to the AZF region there are genes involved in the determination of stature.

1. Bhasin, S., de Kretser, D.M. and Baker, H.W.G. (1994). Pathophysiology and natural history of male infertility. *J. Clin. Endocrinol. Metab.*, 79(6), 1525
2. Palmer, M.S., Sinclair, A.H. and Berta, A.P. (1989). Genetic evidence that ZFY is not the testis determining factor. *Nature*, 342, 937
3. Vollrath, D., Foote, S. and Hilton, A. (1992). The human Y chromosome: A 43 interval map based on natural occuring deletions. *Science*, 258, 52

Related subjects: azoospermia factor, testis determining factor

Y CHROMOSOME, ABNORMALITIES

XX male

Male phenotype and gender, but azoospermic. Small firm testicles, hypospadia and elevated gonadotropins are present. The incidence is 1 in 20 000. Both autosomal recessive and sporadic inheritence are reported. Etiology includes translocation of SRY to an X- or to an autosomal chromosome. Presence of SRY but lack of azoospermia factor accounts for testicular and male sexual differentiation but no initiation of spermatogenesis.

45X/46XY mixed gonadal dysgenesis

Phenotypic male or female with a testis on one side and streak gonad on the other. Sex assignment is usually made according to the degree of virilization. Two-thirds are being raised as females. The testes is often located intra-abdominally and should be removed except where scrotal positioning is possible and the assigned sex is male.

XY azoospermic male

Possibly due to loss of the chromosomal segment Yq containing the azoospermia factor, dicentric Y, rings, etc.

Specific defects affecting the azoospermia factor

Deletions in the Y chromosome may disrupt the the azoospermia factor gene. It is suggested that 10% of azoospermic men have microdeletions of the Y affecting the azoospermia factor.

1. Chandley, A.C., Ambros, P. and McBeath, S. (1986). Short arm dicentric Y chromosome with associated statural defects in a sterile man. *Hum. Genet.*, 73, 350

2. Jaffe, T.H. and Oates, R.D. (1994). Genetic abnormalities and reproductive failure. *Urol. Clin. N. Am.*, 21(3), 395

3. Nagafuchi, S., Namiki, M. and Nakahori, Y. (1993). A minute deletion of the Y chromosome in men with azoospermia. *J. Urol*, 150, 155

4. Takihara, H., Tsukahara, M. and Baba, Y. (1993). Dicentric Y chromosome in azoospermic males. *Br. J. Urol.*, 71, 596

5. Schweikert, H.U., Weissbach, L. and Leyendecker, G. (1982). Clinical, endocrinological and cytological characterization of two 46, XX males. *J. Clin. Endocrinol. Metab.*, 54, 745

Related subjects: azoospermia factor, gonadal dysgenesis, gonadodysgenesis, Y chromosome

YOUNG'S SYNDROME

This is one of the syndromes in which an association of sinopulmonary abnormality and infertility are present. Others syndromes are the immotile cilia syndrome and cystic fibrosis. In patients with Young's syndrome no mutations of the cystic fibrosis gene were found and the pulmonary symptoms (usually bronchiectasy) are mild. In about 50% of affected men the vas deferens is obstructed by abnormal secretions causing azoospermia. Often the epididymal head is distended, possibly due to impaired sperm transport.

1. Handelsmann, D.J., Conway, A.J., Boylan, L.M. and Turtle, J.R. (1984). Young's syndrome: obstructive azoospermia and chronic sinopulmonary infections. *N. Engl. J. Med.*, 310, 3

2. LeLannou, D., Jezequel, P., Blayau, M., Dorval, I., Lemoine, P., Dabadie, A., Roussey, M., Lemarec, B. and Legall, J.Y. (1995). Obstructive azoospermia with agenesis of vas deferens or with bronchiectasia (Young's syndrome), a genetic approach. *Hum. Reprod.*, 10(2), 338

3. Young, D. (1970). Surgical treatment of male infertility. *J. Reprod. Fertil.*, 23, 541

Related subjects: azoospermia, cystic fibrosis, immotile cilia syndrome

Zz

ZINC

Numerous biological mechanisms such as immunity, action of hormones and enzymes (more than 200) are known to be zinc dependent. Leydig cell synthesis of testosterone depends on adequate dietary intake of zinc. Deficiency may affect testicular steroidogenesis and cause testicular failure. Usually seminal zinc level is considered to be an index of prostatic function. Its role in seminal plasma, however, is not clear. Short-term depletion of zinc causes decrease in semen volume and serum testosterone, but other sperm parameters are unchanged. In the literature there is no consensus regarding the relation of seminal zinc levels and sperm density and motility in men with normal and abnormal semen analysis.

1. Carreras, A. and Mendoza, C. (1990). Zinc levels in seminal plasma of fertile and infertile men. *Andrologia*, 22(3), 279

2. Hunt, C.D., Johnson, P.E., Herbel, J.L. and Mullen, L.K. (1992). Effects of dietary zinc depletion on seminal volume and zinc loss, serum testosterone concentrations, and sperm morpholgy in young men. *Am. J. Clin. Nutr.*, 56, 148

3. Xu, B., Chia, S.E., Tsakok, M. and Ong, C.N. (1993). Trace elements in blood and seminal plasma and their relationship to sperm quality. *Reprod. Toxicol.*, 7(6), 613

Related subjects: alcohol, cigarette smoking, nutritional deficiencies, prostate, renal failure, semen analysis — biochemical test of seminal plasma, sickle cell disease

ZONA-DRILLING (ZD)

A form of micromanipulation in which a small hole is made in the zona pellucida, either by digestion with acid Tyrode's media, or mechanically by fine needle or laser. Originally the technique was developed to facilitate the entrance of spermatozoa into the oocyte. Poor fertilization rates and a relative high incidence of polyspermy, together with the improved results of other techniques (especially for intracytoplasmic sperm injection), are responsible for the fact that it has been largely abandoned. Presently, the technique is employed to improve implantation rates of embryos, in which case the method is called assisted hatching.

1. Cohen, J. (1991). Assisted hatching of human embryos. *J. In Vitro Fertil. Embryo Transfer*, 8, 179

2. Gordon, J.W. and Talansky, B.E. (1986). Assisted fertilization by zona drilling: a mouse model for correction of oligospermia. *J. Exp. Zool.*, 239, 347

3. Obruca, A., Strohmer, H., Sakkas, D., Menezo, Y., Kogosowski, A., Barak, Y. and Feichtinger, W. (1994). Use of lasers in assisted fertilization and hatching. *Hum. Reprod.*, 9(9), 1723

Related subjects: micromanipulation

ZONA-FREE HAMSTER EGG PENETRATION TEST

This test assesses the ability of human spermatozoa to undergo capacitation and acrosome reaction, to penetrate the oolemma of the zona-denuded hamster oocyte and to fuse with the oocyte. It provides no information about zona binding and zona penetration. Sensitivity and specificity of the test are such that it cannot discriminate fertile from infertile men, especially in patients with impaired semen parameters. The reason for this is that too many variables are are involved in performing the test itself, as well as in the applied technique between different laboratories.

1. Aitken, J.(1994). On the future of the hamster oocyte penetration assay. *Fertil. Steril.*, 62, 17

2. Cohen, J., Weber, R.F., van der Vijver, J.C. and Zeilmaker, G.H. (1982). *In vitro* fertilizing capacity of human spermatozoa with the use of zona-free hamster ova: interassay variation and prognostic value. *Fertil. Steril.*, 37(4), 565

3. Margalioth, E.J., Feinmesser, M., Navot, D., Mordel, N. and Bronson, R.A. (1989). The long-term predictive value of the zona-free hamster ova sperm penetration assay. *Fertil. Steril.*, 52, 490

4. Muller, C.H., Zarutski, P.W., Stenchever, M.A. and Soules, M.R. (1990). The sperm penetration assay: one of the best methods we have. *Obstet. Gynecol. Rep.*, 2, 412

Related subjects: sperm function tests

ZYGOTE INTRAFALLOPIAN TRANSFER (ZIFT)

An advanced form of assisted reproductive technique where fertilized oocytes in the zygote phase are placed into the Fallopian tube. It combines theoretically the advantages of gamete intrafallopian transfer (physiological milieu for early embryonic development) with those of *in vitro* fertilization (controlled fertilization conditions). The transfer can be performed laparoscopically or transcervically. As with gamete intrafallopian transfer, prospective randomized studies for ZIFT do not show better results than *in vitro* fertilization with intrauterine embryo transfer.

1. Amso, N.N. and Shaw, R.W. (1993). A critical appraisal of assisted reproduction techniques. *Hum. Reprod.*, 8, 168

2. Devroey, P., Braeckmans, P. and Smitz, J. (1986). Pregnancy after translaparoscopic zygote intrafallopian transfer in a patient with with sperm antibodies. *Lancet*, i, 1329

3. Jansen, R.P.S., Anderson, J.P. and Sutherland, P.D. (1988). Non-operative embryo transfer to the Fallopian tube. *N. Engl. J. Med.*, 319, 288

Related subjects: assisted reproduction

Index

The words in heavy type appear as entries in the encyclopedia.